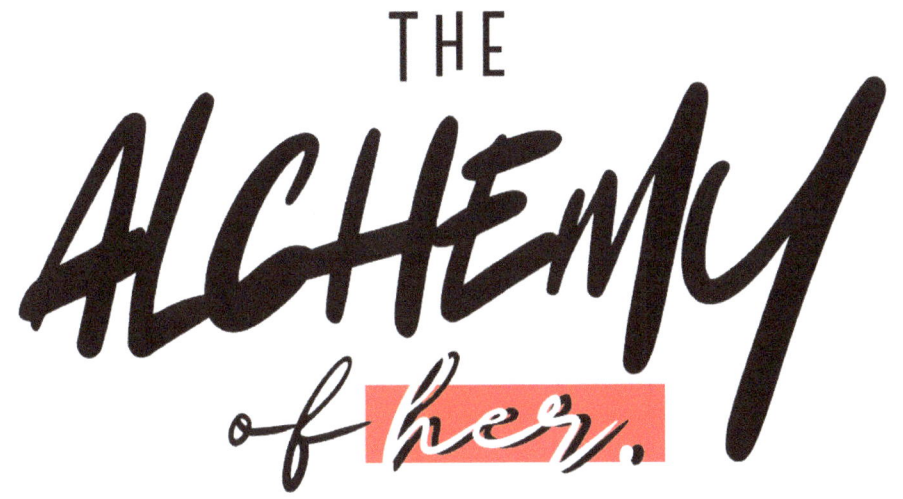

A Holistic Guide to Women's Health, Hygiene, and Reproductive Wellness

BY KIRBY DUNCAN

THE ALCHEMY of her.

SHE'S THE MAGIC, THE MAYHEM & THE MAIN EVENT

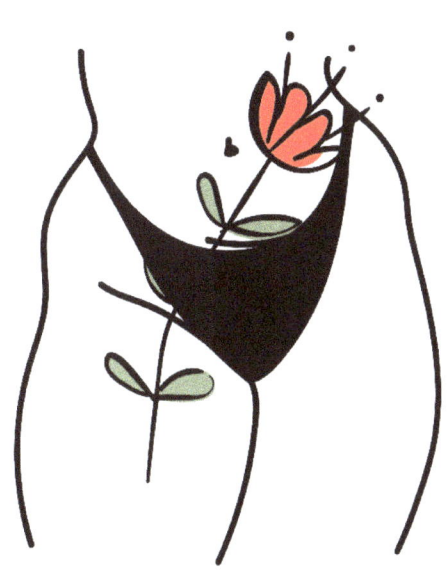

Copyright © 2025 by Kirby Duncan
All rights reserved.

No part of this publication may be reproduced, stored in a retrieval system, or transmitted in any form or by any means – electronic, mechanical, photocopying, recording, or otherwise – without the prior written permission of the publisher, except in the case of brief quotations embodied in critical articles or reviews.

For permissions or inquiries, contact: kirby@yonirx.co

Published by YoniRx™
Printed in the United States of America

First Edition

ISBN: 979-8-218-70362-2 (Paperback)

Cover Design: by Kirby Duncan
Interior Layout: by Kirby Duncan

This book is a work of nonfiction. While every effort has been made to ensure accuracy and integrity, the author accepts no responsibility for errors or omissions.

Disclaimer

The information presented in this book is intended for educational and inspirational purposes only. It is not medical advice. The content is based on the author's personal experience, research, and opinions. The author is not a licensed medical professional. You should always consult a qualified healthcare provider before making changes to your health, wellness, or lifestyle practices.

To my mother, Joyce, who was taken from me by ovarian cancer before I reached womanhood.

Though she didn't have the chance to teach me much about feminine care, her journey has taught me everything about why it matters.

This book is for her. For every woman who wasn't given the knowledge she deserved, and for those who will rise because of it.

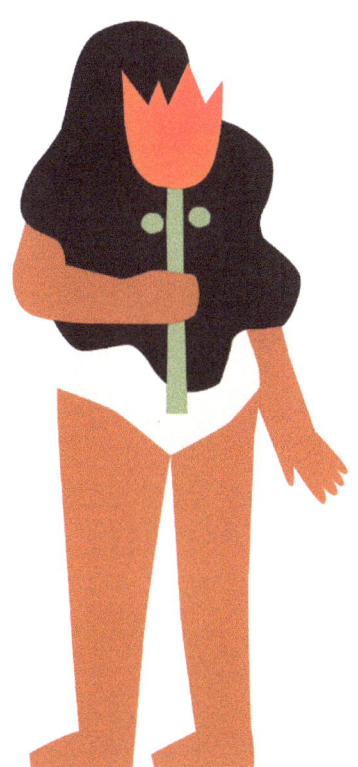

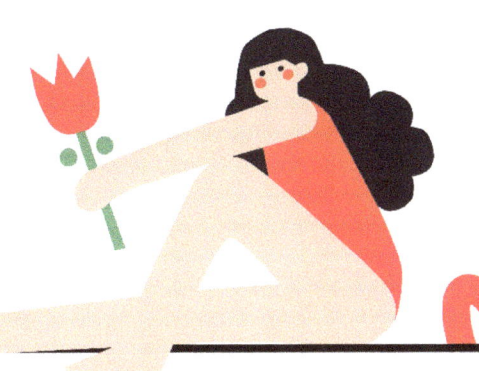

She is made of earth and ember, soft as petals, fierce as fire. She is the keeper of forgotten rituals, the weaver of unseen threads. In her, old wisdom stirs, new light rises—alchemy in motion—turning every wound into wisdom, and every whisper to power. The ordinary dissolves, and the sacred takes shape. She does not seek magic—she is magic.

THE contents

01 WELCOME TO WOMANHOOD — 17

02 THE HORMONAL SYMPHONY — 23

03 HEY, AUNT FLOW — 31

04 MEET YOUR MICROBIOME — 39

05 TURNED ON & TUNED IN — 53

06 WOMB SERVICE — 97

07 MANAGING THE UNMANAGABLE — 111

08 THE GREAT PAUSE — 125

09 TRUST YOUR GUT — 143

10 THE BEAUTY BLUEPRINT — 151

11 THE BARE NECESSITIES — 165

12 STRESS? I DON'T KNOW HER — 175

13 FLUSHING OUT THE FUNK — 183

14 HOLISTIC HEALING — 191

15 THE ALCHEMY OF HER — 201

♡ BONUS PAGES — 209

her ANATOMY

The Vulva

- CLITORAL HOOD
- CLITORIS
- URETHRAL OPENING
- LABIA MINORA
- VAGINAL OPENING
- LABIA MAJORA
- PERINEUM

The Uterus

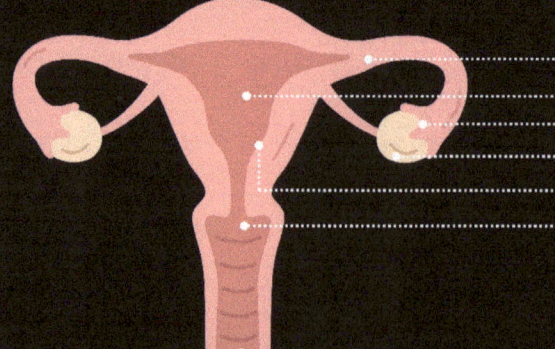

- FALLOPIAN TUBE
- UTERUS
- FIMBRIAE
- OVARY
- ENDOMETRIUM
- CERVIX
- VAGINA (VAGINAL CANAL)

Hey girl. Just curious…

Raise your hand if you thought the vagina was the whole outside part.

Don't worry, no shade. You're not alone, and you're not in trouble. Let's take a moment to meet her anatomy with personality, and purpose. Because every part of her deserves to be seen, understood, and respected. From the vulva to the ovaries.

- Vulva - The whole package. What you see on the outside. Don't call her the vagina—she's got her own name.

- Clitoral Hood - The clit's cute little hoodie. Sometimes she's chillin' underneath.

- Clitoris - She's not shy—she's just waiting for you to learn the map. Do. Not. Skip.

- Urethral Opening - Not where the baby comes out. Not where the penis goes. Just pee, queen.

- Labia Minora (Inner lips) - The delicate petals. Small but mighty—and full of sensation.

- Vaginal Opening - The entrance to the magic portal. She stretches, she cleans herself, she's iconic.

- Labia Majora (Outer lips) - Big sis energy. Protective, plush, and powerful.

- Perineum - The little bridge between front and back.

- Uterus – The OG studio apartment for life. She builds, she sheds, she repeats—monthly.

- Fallopian Tubes – The red carpets for the egg. This is where the meet-up with sperm happens.

- Fimbriae – Flirty fingers at the ends of the tubes. They wave the egg in like 'come on in, girl.'

- Ovaries – The boss babes of hormone and egg production. They're small but in charge.

- Endometrium – Interior decorator of the uterus. Builds a plush lining, then throws it out when no one's moving in (that's your period).

- Cervix – The velvet bouncer. She controls who gets in, and what gets out.

- Vagina – She's the passage, not the whole palace. But she's got power.

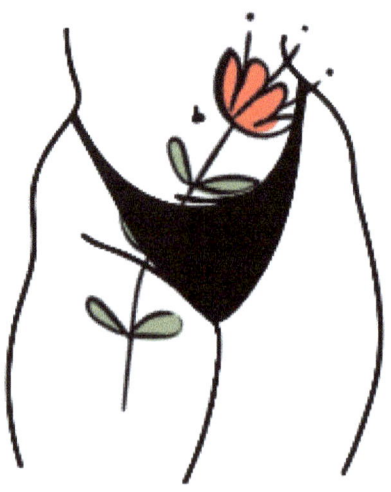

Now that you know her anatomy, let's explore her story.

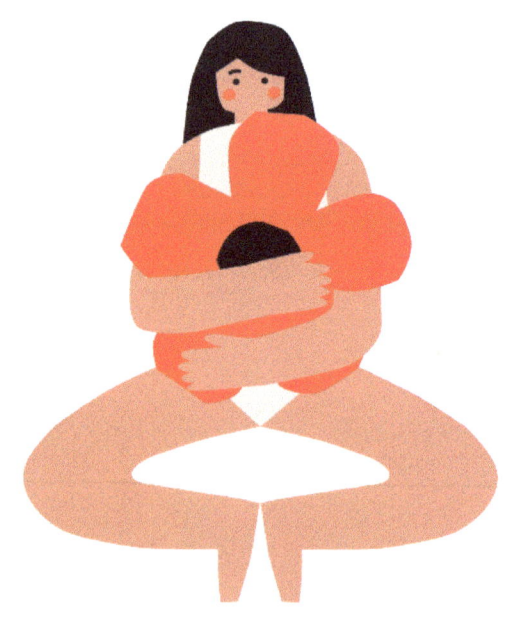

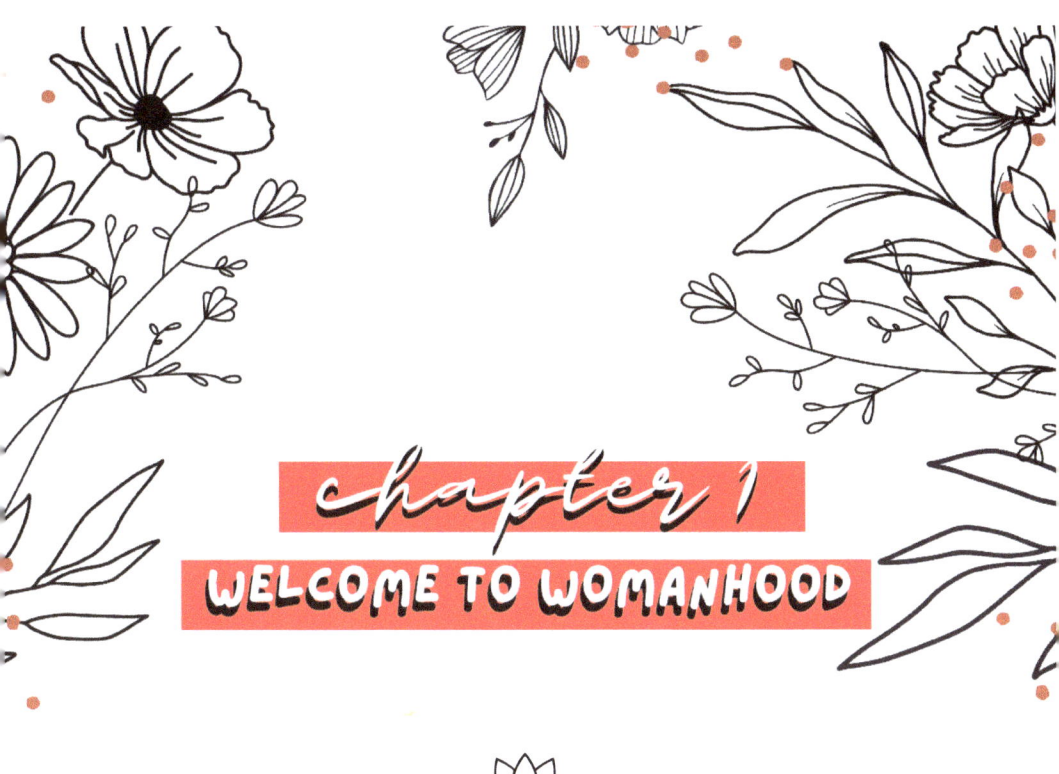

Chapter 1
WELCOME TO WOMANHOOD

Welcome to the grand, chaotic, and awe-inspiring adventure that is being a woman. Whether you've just hit adulthood or have been navigating the hormonal rollercoaster for a while, one thing is certain: your body is a masterpiece of biological brilliance. It bleeds without injury. It adapts to shifting cycles. And if you so choose, it can literally build another human from scratch. No 3D printer required.

While being a woman is magical, it also comes with a lot of fine print. PMS mood swings? Check. Random chin hairs? Check. Cramps that feel like a medieval torture method? Double check. And don't even get me started on the unsolicited health advice from people who think a uterus is a type of dinosaur.

So, before we dive into the nitty-gritty of hormones, microbiomes, and fertility, let's take a moment to appreciate the sheer alchemy of your body. Because once you understand how powerful you are, you'll never take your health for granted again.

Myths You Need to Unlearn

If women's health came with a manual, it would have been written in ten different languages, half in invisible ink, and probably outdated the second you finished reading it. Over the years, we've been fed some questionable advice about our bodies, much of it rooted in outdated science, marketing ploys, or plain old misogyny. Let's debunk a few big ones right now:

"Your period should be exactly 28 days."
Hate to break it to you, but that's a guideline, not a law. Most cycles range from 24 to 35 days, and variation is completely normal. Your body is not a Swiss watch. It's more like a well-loved GPS that occasionally takes scenic detours.

"Painful periods are just part of being a woman."
Nope. While mild discomfort can be normal, debilitating pain isn't. If your period feels like a WWE smackdown, it's time to investigate deeper issues like endometriosis or hormonal imbalances.

"You need to 'clean' your vagina."
Girl, who started this lie? Your vagina is self-cleaning. Douching, scented wipes, and vaginal perfumes are the

equivalent of throwing off the pH balance of an entire ecosystem because you thought it needed a spritz of artificial lavender. Your vagina isn't a Glade plug-in. Leave it alone.

Misinformation about our bodies has been running rampant for centuries, but this book is here to set the record straight. Knowledge is power, and you deserve to wield it like a queen.

Your Hormones, Your Rules

Your hormones are the CEOs of your body. They manage everything from your mood to your metabolism, your libido to your skin health. When they're balanced, you feel like Beyoncé on a good day. When they're out of whack, it's more like an emotional, bloated version of the Hulk with a side of brain fog.

But here's the thing: most of us were never taught how to work with our hormones. Instead, we've been conditioned to suppress, ignore, or medicate them into submission. It's time to change that.

The goal here isn't perfection. It's alignment. When you start working with your body instead of against it, everything changes. More energy. Better moods. Easier periods. And a deep, unshakable appreciation for the body you're in.

The Foundations of Her

Before we get deep into hormones, periods, microbiomes, and all the magic that is womanhood, let's lay down your core foundations. These are the non-negotiables. The daily rituals that hold your hormones, your energy, and your sanity together. You'll see them pop up throughout the book because they matter that much. Consider this your personal cheat code, your survival kit, your "how to human" starter pack.

Hydration

You can't expect your body to run like a queen if you're out here sipping on vibes and dry air. Water is the most basic form of nourishment. Aim for half your body weight in ounces (and yes, add electrolytes if you're feeling fancy). Hormones need hydration. Digestion needs hydration. Glowing skin? Hydration. Period.

Magnesium

This mineral is the quiet hero behind your mood, sleep, muscle recovery, and even pooping. Use magnesium glycinate for relaxation and sleep, and magnesium citrate for digestion. If your jaw is tense, your periods are brutal, or you wake up feeling like a zombie, magnesium is calling your name.

Fiber

Want balanced hormones? Poop daily. Want clearer skin, less bloat, better periods? Fiber, queen. Think flaxseeds, chia, leafy greens, and fruit with the skin on. Fiber helps escort excess estrogen out of the body like a bad date.

Sleep

Not getting enough sleep? Your hormones are already mad at you. Sleep is when your body resets cortisol, produces sex hormones, and repairs everything. Prioritize it like your life depends on it, because honestly, it kind of does.

Movement

You don't need to crush bootcamps to be healthy. Walking, stretching, dancing in the kitchen… all movement counts. Just keep things flowing. Your hormones don't respond well to stagnation (or shame). Keep it joyful, not punishing.

Poop, Sweat, Breathe

These are your detox pathways. Don't neglect them. If you're not pooping, sweating, or breathing deeply, your body is holding on to toxins and stress like emotional baggage. What did Elsa say? Let it go.

So, whenever you're reading a chapter and see these mentioned again and again, just know it's because they're that foundational. We'll always circle back to them because true alchemy doesn't start with fancy supplements or trends. It starts right here.

Now buckle up, because this book is about to take you on a journey through all things womanhood. Unfiltered, unapologetic, and packed with the knowledge you should have been given from the start.

Welcome to *The Alchemy of Her.* Let's get to work.

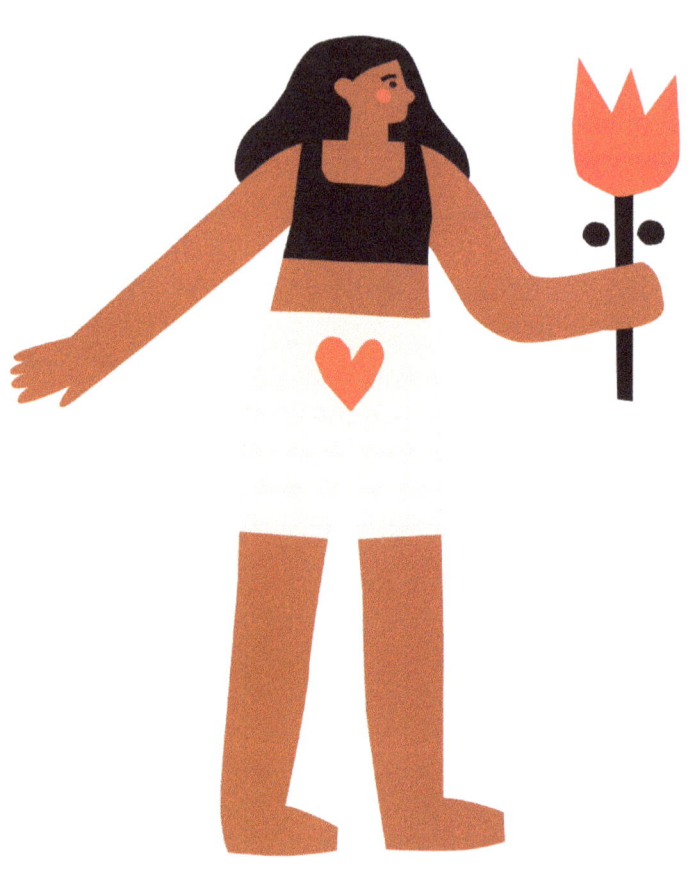

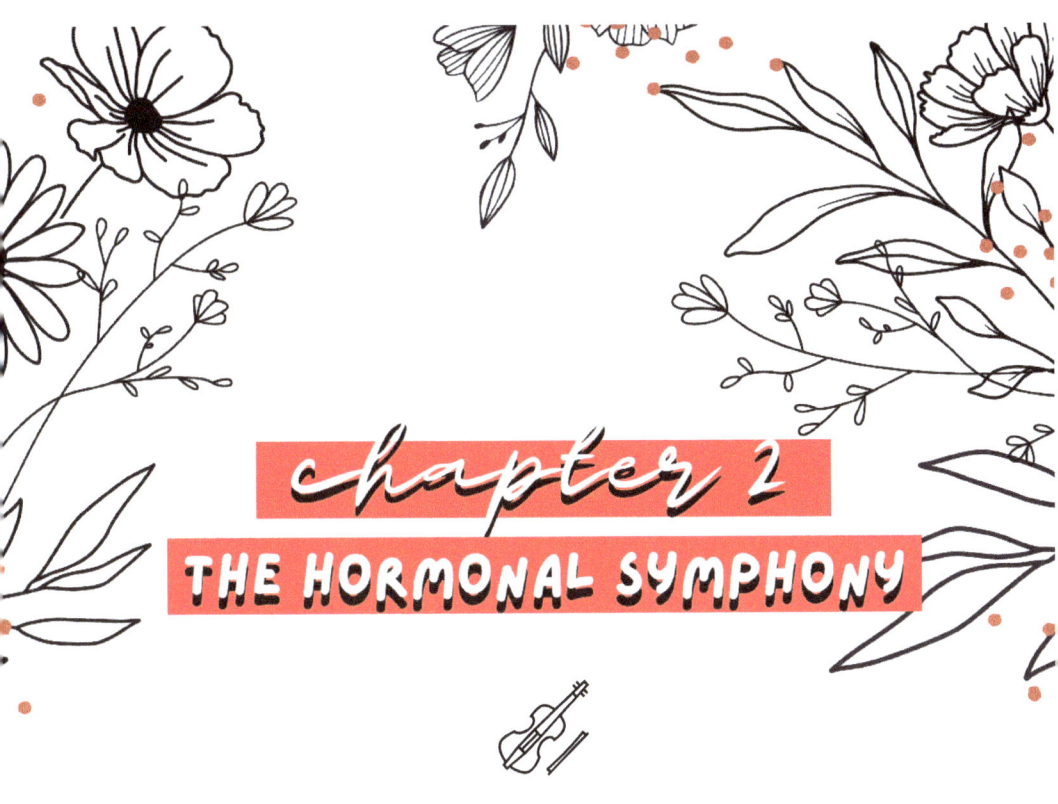

Chapter 2
THE HORMONAL SYMPHONY

Your body isn't just operating on random mood swings and cravings. It's running a full-blown biochemical orchestra, and your hormones are the musicians. When they're in sync, everything flows beautifully. When they're not? It feels like someone gave a toddler a drum set and set it loose inside your nervous system. So what exactly are these hormones, and why do they matter? Let's meet the MVPs.

Estrogen
The queen bee of the reproductive system. She regulates your menstrual cycle, keeps your skin glowing, and even plays a role in brain health. But too much estrogen? Hello, mood swings, bloating, and heavy periods. Too little? Say goodbye to libido and welcome in vaginal dryness.

Progesterone
The calming, grounding best friend to estrogen. This hormone balances out estrogen's chaos and helps with sleep, stress, and period regulation. Low progesterone often means irregular cycles, anxiety, and those awful, tearful PMS meltdowns.

Testosterone
Not just a "guy hormone." Women need testosterone for muscle tone, energy, and a healthy sex drive. Too little and you're exhausted. Too much and you might start seeing unwanted facial hair.

Cortisol
The "fight or flight" hormone. It's great when you're running from danger. Not so great when your body thinks an email from your boss is a life-threatening event. Chronic stress sends cortisol into overdrive, which wrecks your cycle, skin, and metabolism.

Insulin
The blood sugar regulator. Too much sugar, too much stress, or too many processed foods can throw insulin out of whack, leading to weight gain, fatigue, and inflammation.

Thyroid Hormones
The conductors of your body's energy levels. When your thyroid slows down, you feel sluggish, cold, and bloated. When it speeds up, anxiety and weight loss can take over.

Your body works hard to keep these hormones in check, but modern life doesn't make it easy. From stress to processed food to hormone-disrupting chemicals, we're constantly throwing wrenches into our own system. That's why learning to work with your hormones is key.

The Gut-Hormone Connection

What you eat is either fueling your hormonal harmony or throwing it into chaos. Your endocrine system isn't asking for perfection. It just wants some basic respect. Here's how to feed your hormones right.

The Good Stuff

Healthy Fats
Avocados, nuts, seeds, coconut oil, and olive oil help keep hormones balanced and inflammation down. If you've been afraid of fat, it's time to make peace.

Cruciferous Vegetables
Broccoli, cauliflower, Brussels sprouts, and kale help detox excess estrogen and keep your liver happy.

Fiber-Rich Foods
Chia seeds, flaxseeds, lentils, and leafy greens help remove excess hormones and keep digestion smooth.

Protein Power
Grass-fed meat, wild-caught fish, pastured eggs, and plant-based proteins stabilize blood sugar and keep energy levels steady.

Adaptogens
Herbs like maca, ashwagandha, and holy basil help balance stress hormones and support overall well-being.

The Chaos Crew

Sugar Overload
Spikes insulin, fuels inflammation, and sends your hormones on a rollercoaster ride.

Processed Foods
Full of preservatives and additives that mess with your endocrine system.

Dairy (for some people)
Can increase estrogen dominance and trigger acne or bloating. If you love dairy, go organic and grass-fed.

Excess Caffeine and Alcohol
Both can deplete essential nutrients, interfere with sleep, and

spike stress hormones. You don't have to give up coffee—just don't overdo it.

Balancing hormones with food isn't about extreme diets. It's about consistency. The more whole, nutrient-dense foods you add, the better your body functions.

The Holy Trinity of Hormonal Health

Your hormones don't just respond to what you eat. They respond to how you live. Stress, lack of sleep, and neglecting self-care can throw everything off balance.

1. Stress Less

Cortisol is great when you're actually in danger. But if you're constantly in fight-or-flight mode because of work, relationships, or doom scrolling the news, your body is drowning in stress hormones. Chronic cortisol overload can:

- Block progesterone, leading to irregular cycles and PMS
- Disrupt blood sugar, making weight loss nearly impossible
- Wreak havoc on digestion and gut health

Relieve yourself of stress through meditation, breathwork, gentle movement, and saying no to what drains you. Stress management isn't a luxury. It's a necessity.

2. Sleep Like a Queen

Skipping sleep is one of the worst things you can do for your hormones. If you're not sleeping well, your body struggles to:

- Regulate cortisol and insulin, making you crave sugar and caffeine
- Maintain progesterone levels, leading to worse PMS and irregular cycles
- Repair and detox overnight (your liver needs that time to clear out excess hormones)

Go to bed and wake up at the same time daily. Avoid blue light before bed. Try magnesium, chamomile tea, or lavender to help unwind. And yes, the "Sleepy Girl Mocktail" you saw on TikTok actually works.

3. Self-Care

Not all self-care is about bubble baths. Real self-care is about what truly nourishes you.

- Gentle workouts like yoga, Pilates, and walking help balance hormones. Intense exercise during your period can spike cortisol.
- Get out into the sun. Soaking up vitamin D is key for mood and metabolism.
- Hormones love oxytocin—the "feel-good" hormone that's released when you hug someone, laugh, or cuddle a pet. Prioritize connection, even in small ways.

Your body is constantly talking to you. When you feel exhausted, moody, or out of sync, it's not betrayal. It's communication. Learning to listen and respond is one of the most powerful things you can do.

Balancing your hormones isn't about chasing perfection. It's about awareness. Every small shift, what you eat, how you rest, how you breathe matters. Your body is powerful. When you support it with intention, it will meet you with more clarity, more energy, and more peace.

So the question is: are you ready to start working *with* your hormones instead of fighting them?

Your body's already waiting.

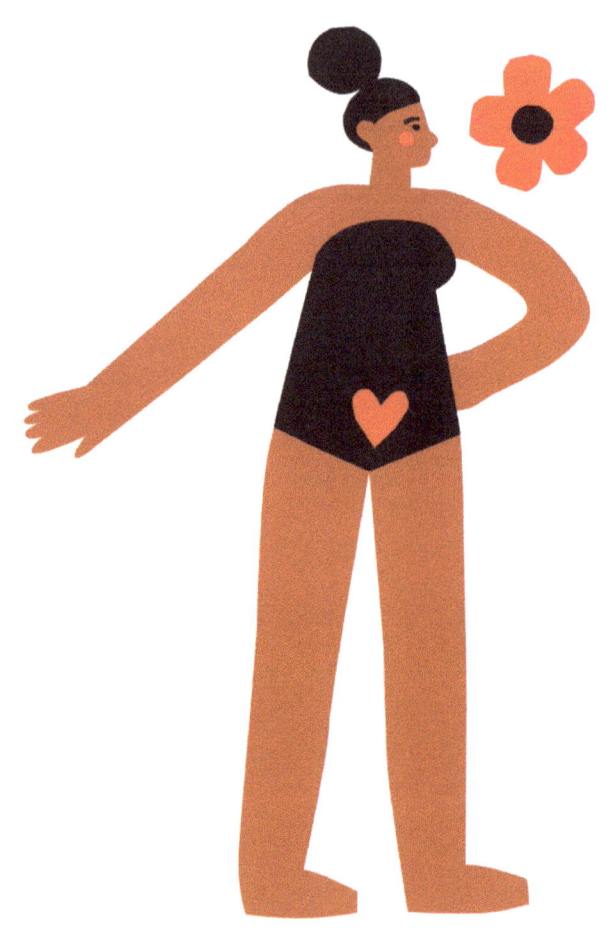

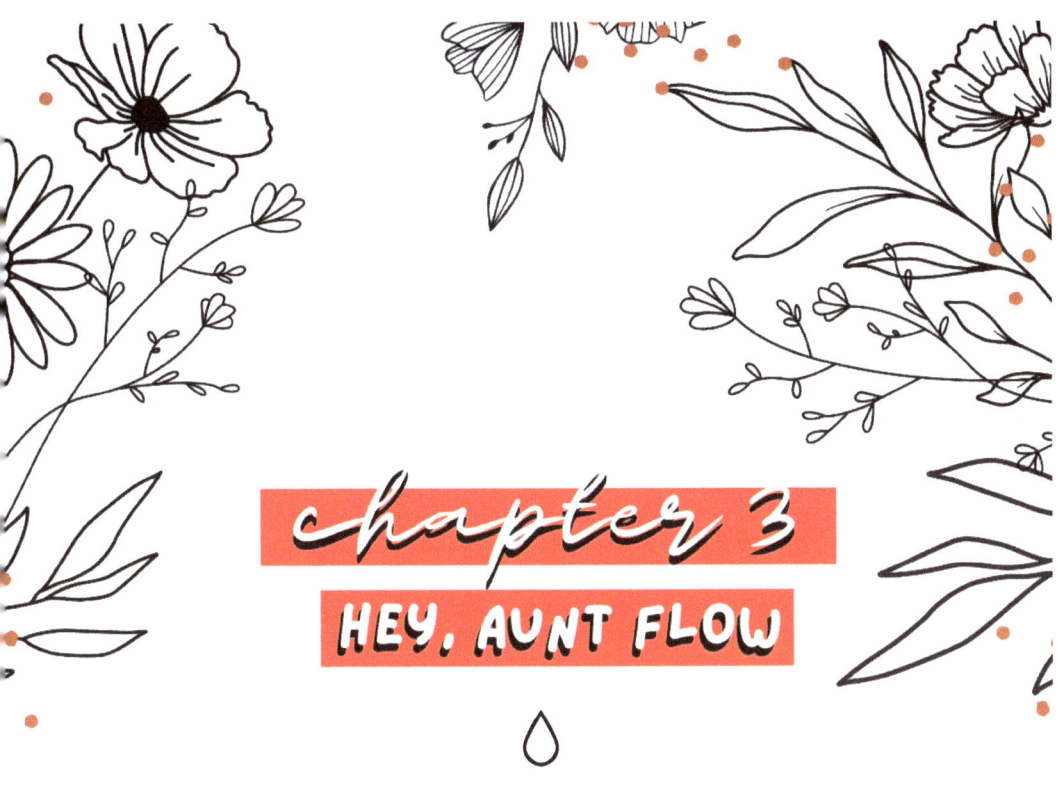

Chapter 3
Hey, Aunt Flow

The menstrual cycle—a monthly reminder that your body is functioning as it should, or a complete and utter nightmare depending on how things are going. Whether your period is a mild inconvenience or an absolute hellscape, understanding what's normal and what's not is the first step toward making peace with your cycle.

What's Normal?

- Cycle length between 24-35 days (because, contrary to popular belief, not every woman's cycle is a perfect 28 days).

- Mild cramping that doesn't leave you curled up like a shrimp.

- Blood color ranging from bright red to deep maroon (because your uterus isn't a Pinterest aesthetic).
- Flow lasting anywhere from 3-7 days (again, variation is normal).

- Some mild bloating, breast tenderness, or mood shifts before your period.

What's Not Normal?

- Pain so bad you can't function. If you need to cancel plans, pop painkillers like candy, or contemplate selling your uterus on the black market, something isn't right. This could be a sign of endometriosis, adenomyosis, or hormonal imbalances.

- Extremely heavy bleeding. If you're soaking through a pad or tampon every hour or passing large clots, this isn't just a "bad period"—it could be a sign of fibroids, hormonal imbalances, or other underlying issues.

- Irregular cycles (consistently). It's normal for your cycle to fluctuate a bit, but if your period goes MIA for months at a time or shows up twice a month uninvited, it's time to investigate.

- Severe PMS that makes you feel like an unhinged villain. If you experience debilitating anxiety, depression, rage, or extreme fatigue before your period, you might have PMDD (premenstrual dysphoric disorder) or progesterone imbalance.

If your period is making your life miserable, it's not something to "just deal with." Painful, irregular, or excessively heavy periods are not normal, and you don't have to suffer in silence. Your body is trying to tell you something. Time to listen.

Period Products

With all the modern advancements in period care, why does it still feel like a battlefield every month? Because not all period products are created equal. Let's break them down so you can choose the best option for your body and flow.

Tampons: The Classic Option

Pros: Convenient, discreet, and effective for most flows.

Cons: Conventional tampons contain bleach, dioxins, and synthetic fibers that can disrupt vaginal health. Also, leaving them in too long (*hello, Toxic Shock Syndrome!*) is *not* an option.

Tip: If you love tampons, opt for 100% organic \cotton to avoid unnecessary chemicals.

Change every 4-8 hours, max. If your tampon is fully saturated in under 2 hours, you may have a heavy flow and should size up or switch to a more absorbent method. NEVER leave a tampon in over night.

Pads: The Safe, No-Fuss Option

Pros: No risk of TSS, easy to use, and great for overnight protection.

Cons: Can feel bulky, messy, sometimes lead to chafing, and many conventional pads contain plastic and synthetic fragrances (*which your vagina does not* need).

Tip: Go for organic, non-toxic pads or try cloth pads if you want an eco-friendly option.

Change every 4-6 hours, depending on flow. If you're waking up in a bloodbath at 2am, it's time to use a more absorbent pad for nighttime.

Menstrual Cups: The Game-Changer

Pros: Cost-effective, eco-friendly, and can last up to 12 hours without leaks.

Cons: Takes some practice to insert/remove (*but once you get it, it's a game-changer*).

Tip: Make sure you sterilize your cup between cycles. Your vagina deserves cleanliness, not last month's leftovers.

Can be worn for up to 12 hours, but for heavier flows, empty and rinse every 5-6 hours to prevent leaks and discomfort. Always sanitize between cycles with a mild, unscented soap, or even boiling water.

Period Underwear: The Ultimate Convenience

Pros: No leaks, super comfortable, and great for lighter flow days.

Cons: Can be expensive, and you'll need a few pairs to get through your cycle.

Tip: Look for period underwear with moisture-wicking fabric to avoid that *damp diaper* feeling. Rinse in cold water before tossing into the wash - hot water can set stains.

Change every 8-12 hours or as needed, depending on absorbency. If it starts to feel damp, time to swap.

What Not to Use

- Scented pads and tampons. If your vagina needed perfume, it would have come with a built-in fragrance diffuser.

- Douching. Your vagina cleans itself—don't mess with her ecosystem.

- Leaving tampons in for more than 8 hours. Seriously, let's not play Russian roulette with toxic shock syndrome.

Your period products should work *for* you, not against you. Choose what makes you feel comfortable, safe, and in control of your cycle.

Syncing with Your Cycle

Your menstrual cycle isn't just about bleeding, it's a four-phase hormonal blueprint that affects your energy, mood, metabolism, and even how social you feel. Learning how to work with your cycle instead of fighting against it can change *everything*.

Phase 1: Menstrual Phase (Days 1-5ish)
What's Happening: Hormones are at their lowest. Your uterus is shedding its lining.

How You Feel: Tired, introspective, needing snacks and quiet.

Best Activities:
- Rest. Seriously. You're shedding an organ.
- Gentle movements like stretching or walking

- Journaling or goal reflection

What to Eat: Warm, iron-rich foods like soup, bone broth, lentils, and spinach.

Phase 2: Follicular Phase (Days 6-14ish)
What's Happening: Estrogen rises. Energy returns.

How You Feel: Creative, focused, social.

Best Activities:
- High-energy workouts
- Big projects or brainstorming
- Trying new things

What to Eat: Lean proteins, healthy carbs (quinoa, sweet potatoes), and fermented foods for gut support.

Phase 3: Ovulation (Days 14-17ish)
What's Happening: Estrogen peaks. You're most fertile (take note, even if you're not trying to get pregnant).

How You Feel: Confident, radiant, magnetic.

Best Activities:
- Public speaking, social events, networking
- Intense workouts
- Date nights or intimacy

What to Eat: Zinc-rich foods like pumpkin seeds or oysters, hydrating fruits, and anti-inflammatory meals.

Phase 4: Luteal Phase (Days 18-28ish)
What's Happening: Progesterone rises. Your body prepares for a possible pregnancy.

How You Feel: Slower, maybe moody or sensitive.

Best Activities:
- Low-impact movements like walking or Pilates
- Finishing tasks and checking things off
- Setting boundaries and staying grounded

What to Eat: Magnesium-rich foods like dark chocolate, leafy greens, and nuts.

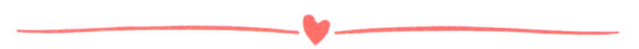

Your period isn't just something to "get through"—it's a blueprint for better health, productivity, and self-awareness. The more you learn to work with your cycle, the easier (and dare I say, more empowering) it becomes. So, let's stop seeing our periods as the enemy. Your body is on your side; you just have to start listening.

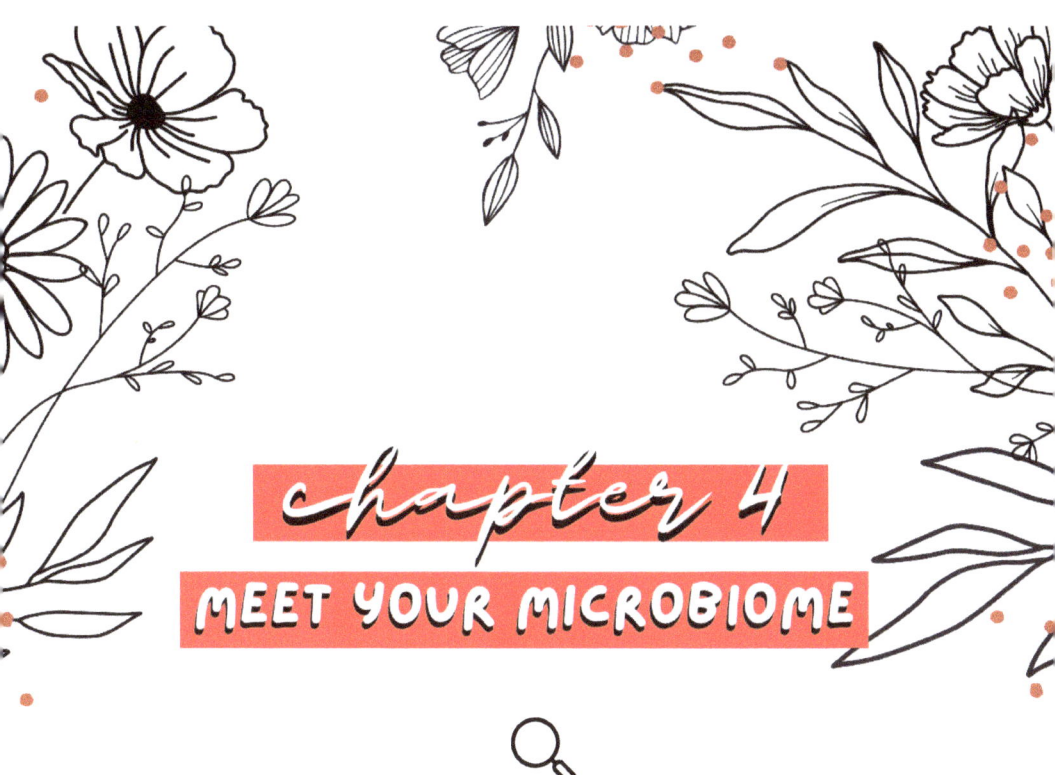

Chapter 4
MEET YOUR MICROBIOME

Your vagina is a self-cleaning, pH-regulating, bacteria-balancing queen. It's an entire ecosystem that works tirelessly to protect you from infections, maintain moisture, and keep everything running smoothly. But like any ecosystem, it's delicate. One wrong move (or one poorly chosen product) can throw it into chaos faster than you can say "yeast infection."

Meet Your Microbiome

Inside your vagina lives a thriving community of bacteria, mostly Lactobacillus, the good guys responsible for keeping everything in balance. They:

- Maintain an acidic pH (between 3.8 and 4.5) to keep harmful bacteria and yeast in check
- Produce lactic acid and hydrogen peroxide to fight off infections

- Work as your first line of defense against BV, yeast infections, and UTIs

But when things go south? That's when you get itching, burning, discharge changes, and the dreaded off smell that makes you side-eye your underwear.

Microbiome Disruptors

Let's shine a light on the most common culprits and their triggers.

Urinary Tract Infections (UTIs)
Caused when bacteria, often E. coli, sneak into the urinary tract. You'll notice burning when you pee, frequent urges to go, and cloudy or smelly urine.

Yeast Infections
An overgrowth of Candida leads to itching, redness, and thick discharge that looks like cottage cheese.

Bacterial Vaginosis (BV)
An imbalance in your vaginal bacteria. Symptoms often include a fishy odor and grayish discharge. Some people have no symptoms at all but still experience disruption.

Common Triggers

Douching & Scented Products
The biggest scam ever. Your vagina cleans itself, and douching wipes out the good bacteria while giving harmful bacteria a VIP pass to take over.

Antibiotics
Sometimes necessary, but they don't just kill bad bacteria; they also wipe out the good ones, leaving your microbiome vulnerable.

Hormonal Imbalances
Estrogen plays a role in vaginal flora, and when it's off (thanks, birth control or stress), your microbiome suffers.

High Sugar Diet & Processed Foods
Sugar feeds yeast and bad bacteria, making infections more likely.

Unprotected Sex & Semen Exposure

Semen has a higher pH (7-8), which can disrupt your vaginal acidity and throw off your flora.

Wearing Tight, Non-Breathable Underwear
Your vagina needs airflow. Trapping moisture down there is a yeast infection's dream come true.

Your vagina is not high maintenance—it just doesn't tolerate disrespect.

Avoiding a Microbiome Meltdown

If you've ever had BV, a yeast infection, or a UTI, you know that once your microbiome is off, it takes real effort to get things back to normal. Here's how to prevent (and fix) a microbiome meltdown.

1. Keep It Clean, But Not Too Clean

- Wash with water and mild, unscented soap (if needed). No fragrances, no harsh surfactants, no foam parties.

- Let her breathe. Cotton underwear > synthetic fabrics. At night, consider going commando.

2. Support your pH and your flora

- Probiotics are your friend. Look for ones with Lactobacillus rhamnosus and Lactobacillus reuteri (these strains are best for vaginal health). Probiotic-rich foods include yogurt, kimchi, sauerkraut, and kefir help replenish your microbiome. Eating yogurt during and after a round of antibiotics is some real self-love.

- Use pH-friendly intimate care. If you must use wipes or washes, make sure they're pH-balanced to 3.8-4.5.

- Rethink your lube. Some lubricants have ingredients (like glycerin) that feed yeast. Choose a natural, pH-balanced lube instead.
- Limit sugar & processed foods. Sugar feeds yeast, which can make infections more frequent.

- Drink plenty of water. Hydration keeps vaginal tissues healthy and flushes out toxins.

4. Be Smart About Sex & Hygiene

- Always pee after sex to flush out potential bacteria that could creep up into your urethra and cause a UTI.

- Avoid using spit as lube. Just…no. It introduces bacteria from your mouth into your vagina, and that's a recipe for

an infection. That said, please be mindful of your partner's oral health. If they have poor oral hygiene or gum disease (which is common), that bacteria can disrupt your vaginal microbiome. (*A clean mouth = a happy vagina*).
- Also worth noting: oral sex can also introduce imbalances. The mouth has its own microbiome—and if it's out of balance, it can mess with yours. Let's just say: floss, brush, and maybe rethink that late-night fast food before foreplay.

Your vaginal microbiome works 24/7 to protect you.
Treat her well, and she'll return the favor.

Bacterial Ping-Pong

If you keep getting BV or yeast infections after treatment, don't blame your body. Blame the loop.

Male partners can carry BV-associated bacteria in their urethra or under the foreskin without ever showing symptoms. That means you can treat it, feel better, and then boom—back again after sex. It's not your hygiene. It's the bacterial ping-pong.

 If you're in a relationship or frequently having sex with the same partner, it's worth considering partner treatment. This may mean antibiotics (like metronidazole or clindamycin), and yes, even if he "feels fine."

Probiotics, Prebiotics, and pH

So, we've established that your vaginal health is largely bacteria dependent. The key to a healthy, balanced vagina is probiotics, prebiotics, and maintaining the right pH. Let's go into more detail.

Probiotics

Taking oral probiotics or using vaginal suppositories with Lactobacillus strains can help:

- Restore healthy bacteria after antibiotics or infections.
- Prevent yeast infections, BV, and UTIs.
- Improve vaginal moisture and overall comfort

Best probiotic strains for vaginal health:

Lactobacillus rhamnosus (protects against BV and UTIs).

Lactobacillus reuteri (balances pH and supports vaginal flora).

Lactobacillus crispatus (helps keep your vaginal microbiome acidic).

Prebiotics

Probiotics need food to thrive, and that's where prebiotics come in. These fiber-rich foods help good bacteria flourish:

- Garlic
- Onions
- Bananas
- Asparagus
- Flaxseeds

A diet rich in prebiotic foods supports not just your gut, but your vaginal microbiome too.

pH Balance

Your vagina is naturally acidic for a reason — it kills off harmful bacteria and yeast. If your pH creeps too high (above 4.5), BV and yeast infections become more likely.

Infection Prevention Cheat Sheet

Urinary Tract Infections (UTIs)

1. Hydrate - Drinking plenty of water flushes bacteria out.
2. Cranberry Juice - May prevent bacteria from sticking to urinary tract walls.

3. Wipe Front to Back – Prevents bacteria from migrating where they shouldn't.
4. Pee After Sex – Helps clear out bacteria before it causes problems.

Bacterial Vaginosis (BV)

1. Skip the Scents – No scented soaps, douches, or vaginal deodorants. They mess up your flora.
2. Take Probiotics – Consuming probiotics may help maintain a healthy vaginal microbiome.
3. Safe Sex Practices – Using condoms and cleaning sex toys reduces the risk of BV.

Yeast Infections

1. Stay Dry – Change out of wet clothes ASAP. Yeast thrives in moisture.
2. Choose Breathable Fabrics – Cotton underwear = more airflow. Give her some air at night.
3. Mind Your Diet – Limit sugar, because yeast feeds on it.

Let's Talk STI's & STD's

We've talked a lot about infections that come from inside—like BV, yeast, or UTIs. The kind that happen when your pH is off, your microbiome is stressed, or your hormones are doing the most. But STIs? That's a different lane.

STIs don't come from your bath soap, leggings, or skipped probiotics. They come from sex. From another person's body entering yours—and whatever bacteria, viruses, or imbalances they bring along with them. And here's the thing: you can't always feel them. They don't always show symptoms. Sometimes they live quietly in your body for weeks, months, even years. Which is why testing and awareness matter—not fear, not shame. Just facts.

So let's clear up the difference between STIs and STDs, how they show up, how to protect yourself, and how to stay in control of your sexual health. Because the goal isn't just to have sex—it's to have sex that doesn't leave you with a surprise prescription or a pelvic floor therapist on speed dial.

STIs vs. STDs

STI (Sexually Transmitted Infection)
An infection that's been transmitted but hasn't necessarily caused symptoms yet.

STD (Sexually Transmitted Disease)
When an STI causes noticeable symptoms or complications.

In other words, all STDs start as STIs—but not all STIs become full-blown diseases. And many people don't even know they're infected, which is how things spread so quickly. Especially if they've never been tested.

How Long Do STIs Take to Show Up?

Each infection has its own "window period" (how long it takes to show symptoms or appear on a test):

- Chlamydia & Gonorrhea: 1-3 weeks
- Trichomoniasis: 5-28 days
- Syphilis: 3 weeks - 3 months
- HIV: Up to 3 months (but most accurate at 4-6 weeks)
- Herpes (HSV): 2-12 days (but not everyone gets obvious sores)
- HPV: Can take months or even years to show up as warts or abnormal pap smears

Moral of the story? Symptoms are not a reliable guide. Testing is.

How Often Should You Get Tested?

Let's keep it simple:

- If you're sexually active with multiple partners: every 3-6 months

- New partner? Test before and again 2-3 weeks after (depending on window periods)

- If your partner has other partners, or you're unsure of their status: test more often

- If you have symptoms, even mild: test now

And don't forget oral and anal sex count too—ask for throat and rectal swabs if applicable.

STI Prevention: Not Just Condoms

- Condoms and dental dams lower risk but don't protect against everything (HPV, herpes can be passed through skin-to-skin contact).

- Get tested every 3-6 months if you're sexually active with multiple partners.

- Don't rely on someone else's test results unless you saw the paperwork *and* the date.

- Limit partners who are untested, casual, or don't prioritize protection.

- And *please* avoid douching—it wipes out your good bacteria and leaves your microbiome vulnerable

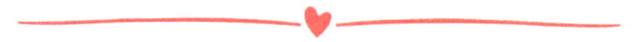

Your vaginal microbiome isn't asking for perfection, just respect. She's not high maintenance, but she is sensitive. And she's tired of being thrown off by pH killers, careless partners, and that one soap that smells like a tropical smoothie but acts like bleach.

When you support her with intention—protecting her ecosystem, honoring her rhythms, and choosing partners who care about your health, too—she shows up for you in the best ways: fewer infections, more natural lubrication, easier cycles, and a body that feels safe to live in.

Your vagina is not a problem to be managed. She's a whole ecosystem worth protecting. Treat her like the queen she is and she'll protect your throne right back.

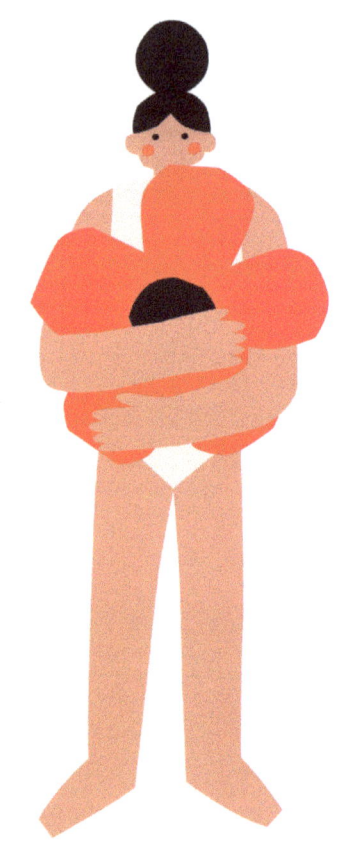

chapter 5
TURNED ON & TUNED IN

Alright, ladies—a whole chapter dedicated to orgasms and sexual reclamation? Say less. When you think "*The Alchemy of Her*" is this where your mind led you? While there is so much depth to being a woman, understanding and achieving pleasure may be the hardest equation of them all.

We're going deeper than "just have a glass of wine and relax." This is about reclaiming your sensual self—not for anyone else, but for you. We'll talk about how to taste like a smoothie, get wetter without synthetic shortcuts, and make orgasms happen without needing a NASA-level strategy. This is going to be a long one. So, whether your libido has ghosted you completely or you're just craving more confidence, awareness, and pleasure in your body, this chapter is for you. Let's get into it.

You Deserve This Feeling

Before we dive deep into everything orgasm –positions, G-spots, size myths, even backdoor bliss–I want to pause right here and acknowledge something important:

If talking and thinking about your pleasure feels foreign, taboo, overwhelming, or even "too much" … that's okay. You're undoing years of conditioning that told you to shrink, please others, and feel shame about your own body. So yeah, it might feel big. It might feel scary. But that doesn't mean it's wrong. It means it's real. And it's yours.

You don't have to earn your orgasm. You don't have to be "good enough," or relaxed enough, or in a relationship to deserve one. You don't even need anyone else in the room. Your orgasm is a holy reminder that you are alive.

And while we're here, let me just say it… Your orgasm might indeed be more powerful, deeper, and longer-lasting than a man's. Not out of competition. But because you are wired for depth. For waves. For surges. For birth. Let your body show you what she's been holding all along. This is true alchemy.

The Mind-Body Connection

Your brain is your biggest sex organ. You could be in the perfect position, with the perfect partner, and the perfect playlist and still feel nothing if your mind is elsewhere.

Thoughts like:

"Do I look okay from this angle?"
"Did I respond to that email?"
"Wait... is he done already?"

These are orgasm blockers. Full stop. But when you drop into your breath? When you quiet the outside world? When your mind gets turned on? Whew. Whole different game. Erotic audio, visualization, fantasies, affirmations, breathwork, mirror work, meditative masturbation—these are all ways to tune your mind into your body. When they work together, your orgasm becomes less about friction and more about frequency.

The Real Main Character

Let's just say it loud: The clitoris is not optional.
She is not a button to be ignored or pressed like you're refreshing an app. She is the actual main character in most women's orgasms, and yet so many of us were never taught how important she is. Or worse, were taught to feel weird or guilty about touching her.

So, here's a little anatomy love note:

The head of the clitoris has 8,000 nerve endings. More than *any other part of the human body*, including the penis. The penis has about 4,000 nerve endings at the tip. So yes, we're *literally* twice as sensitive.

And get this—what you see on the outside (that lil' pearl) is only the tip. The clitoris is a whole internal structure shaped like a wishbone, wrapping around the vaginal canal. She's deep. She's powerful. She's designed exclusively for pleasure. So if someone's skipping over your clit and diving straight into penetration like they're punching in a timecard, tell them politely (or not-so-politely) to circle back.

And if you're not exploring clitoral pleasure with yourself, girl, meet the Rose. You know the one. The viral little air-pulsing queen that took over the internet and may or may not have summoned ancestors. Use it. Worship your clit. Make eye contact with her in the mirror. Say thank you. Because when you prioritize *her*, your whole body starts remembering how to *feel* again.

What an Orgasm Actually Feels Like

An orgasm isn't just some final destination you're supposed to reach like it's a prize at the end of a treadmill. It's more like a full-body exhale. A spiritual, hormonal & emotional detonation.

It can start as a warmth. A tightness. A pulsing sensation that begins low, deep in your pelvis—or even in your toes—and then spreads like wildfire. You might feel your muscles contract in waves. You might make a sound you've never made before. Your breath might catch. Your legs might shake. Your thoughts might disappear. You might cry. Laugh. Moan. Collapse. Scream. Or go completely still. And guess what? It's all normal. All yours.

Now, how do you know you're getting close? That's when everything in your body starts tightening *and* opening at the same time. There's a tipping point—like being right at the top of a roller coaster—and then? You let go. You *fall* into it. You surrender to the pleasure. That's the part a lot of women accidentally shy away from, because the build-up feels so powerful, it almost scares you. You feel all of that building, and then… nothing. You were right there. Right at the edge. Your body was saying yes. But something inside you whispered no. If that's been happening to you, you're not broken. You're not "doing it wrong." You're just protecting yourself. So many women get *right to the edge* and then something short-circuits. When you get close to orgasm, your body is *surrendering*. It's opening. It's letting go. And if you've ever had to hold it together for survival—emotionally, physically, sexually—that kind of surrender can feel terrifying. Your brain might start scanning for danger, even when you're safe. You might tighten instead of open. You might suddenly feel disconnected or overwhelmed.

That doesn't mean you're broken. It means your body remembers. It means she's cautious. It means she's asking, "Is it okay to let go?"

So start there. Let her know she's safe now. That she's allowed to melt. That no one's rushing her or expecting anything from her. And if you get close and back away? That's still a win. That's still a softening. That's still your body waking up.

Come back to the breath. Slow it down. Let yourself edge without pressure. Let the build be enough. The more you create safety, the more your body will stop bracing for impact and start reaching for release. There's no expiration date on pleasure. No deadline for orgasm. And no shame in taking your time. It's not about chasing a climax. It's about reclaiming your right to *feel*–all the way through.

Can You Really Have Multiple Orgasms?

Uh, yes. Yes, yes, YES.
Unlike men whose orgasms are typically followed by a refractory period (aka nap time) many women can experience back-to-back orgasms with no cool-down required. Because your body doesn't just end after climax. Sometimes she's just getting warmed up. And multiple orgasms don't have to look like fireworks every time. Sometimes they come in gentle waves. Sometimes it's a deep quake followed by smaller, rolling aftershocks. Sometimes the second one is even stronger than the first because you've let go of the pressure. The key?

Stay present. Don't rush away from the moment. Keep riding the wave instead of pulling back. Use breath, sound, movement, or toys to keep the energy flowing. And don't overthink it. Your body knows the way.

The G-Spot

Let's talk about the highly Googled G-spot. You've heard of it. You've hoped for it. Maybe you've even faked meeting it just to wrap things up. No shame, we've all been there. But the G-spot *does* exist, and unlocking it? Baby, that's a whole different kind of chemistry class.

Anatomically speaking (just for a sec, don't zone out on me), the G-spot is usually located about two to three inches inside the vagina, on the front wall, toward your belly button. When aroused, it can feel slightly spongy or ridged, and when stimulated just right, it can unlock toe-curling, breathtaking, mattress-gripping kind of pleasure. But here's the catch: it's not just about location, it's about the damn combination. Angle. Pressure. Rhythm.

Some women can't even feel her unless their legs are perfectly straight and locked like they're planking. Some need to be flat on their back like a crime scene outline, muscles clenched like they're lifting a car off their toddler. Some need to tense every fiber, others need to relax like they just hit a blunt. Some need external stimulation at the same time (because she doesn't do solo acts). And some–*bless y'all*–need to stop breathing

entirely to get there. Your orgasm code is unique. And you're not broken if it takes time to figure it out. This isn't a one-size-fits-all GPS. You might need to try cowgirl leaning forward, missionary with a pillow under your hips, or angled doggy with a deep arch. You might need clitoral stimulation *at the same time*
(because spoiler alert: most women do). You might need lube. You might need complete silence, or a playlist titled "Nasty but Classy." Let your body lead. Let her teach you. Let her stutter, hum, and whisper what works. Because once you find that code? Baby… you're gonna be unlocking pleasure like it's a safe with generational wealth inside. It's giving spiritual awakening. May the odds be ever in your favor.

Now let's break down a few position favorites that help many women get closer to their personal pleasure code:

Pillow Princess (Missionary with Elevation)
Lie flat on your back with a pillow or two under your hips to create a natural tilt toward your G-spot. Great for shallow thrusts and pressure on the front wall. Bonus: you get to just lay there like a goddess while he (or your toy) does the work.

Curl-Forward Cowgirl
You're on top, but leaning *way* forward so your chest is close to their chest or the bed. This angle can create deep contact with your G-spot and allows for that grindy, controlled rhythm that lets *you* take charge of the pressure and pace.

Angled Doggy with a Deep Arch
Classic doggy but with your back deeply arched (not flat). Think "booty popped, spine like a dip." This changes the entry angle and lets the front vaginal wall take center stage.

Spooning with a Slow Grind
Side-lying positions are great for lazy Sundays and gentle but focused pressure. With the right hip tilt, it becomes intimate *and* G-spot savvy.

Chair or Edge Play
Sitting on the edge of a chair, bed, or couch with legs apart can give your partner a straight shot toward the G-spot. Also works great with toys. Stability recommended unless you're okay with falling off mid-climax (some of us are thrill-seekers, I get it).

And if you're still not feeling it? That's okay too. Some women are clitorally dominant, some are cervically sensitive, some are just tired… and all of that is normal. Your pleasure doesn't need to fit into a box, a trend, or a diagram.

Let's Talk Size, Sis

Okay, so while we're decoding orgasms and mapping out the G-spot, let's get real about something that's been causing unnecessary identity crises and performance pressure for decades.

Size.

Now, I'm not here to rain on the "big D energy" parade. If that's your thing, you better ride that roller coaster and scream with pride. But here's the cold, hard, sweet little truth:

As we mentioned earlier, the G-spot is only 2 to 3 inches inside. That's right. Two to three. *Uno, dos, tres.* You don't need a footlong. You don't need a lightsaber. You don't need to rearrange your organs to find pleasure. You need connection, positioning, communication, and sometimes a little elevation. Let me break it down like this: You wouldn't use a sledgehammer to hang a picture frame, right? Same energy. It's not always about the tool, it's about how you use it.

A partner with six inches who knows how to angle, listen, tease, and stay consistent will take you farther than someone with eight inches who's treating your body like a punching bag. Sorry, not sorry.
And girl, if your partner is making you feel like they need to be huge to please you? Run. The real ones ask what you like,

where to go, how to adjust, and learn your rhythm like a favorite song.

Size matters in the sense of what you personally enjoy, but not in the way society has hyped it. Some women feel more full and stimulated with longer or girthier partners. Others get overstimulated and need shallower, focused pressure. Some want the stretch, some want the spot. And all of that is valid. So the next time someone asks, "Does size matter?"
You can smile and say, "Not when you know where the hell you're going and how to drive."

Okay But, Squirting. Is It Pee or…?

Ah yes. The mystery. The myth. The splash zone.
Let's talk about it: squirting, also called female ejaculation.

First, no, it's not "just pee." But also… yes, there might be a *little* bit of pee mixed in. Squirting usually comes from stimulation of the G-spot. When stimulated, some people release a clear to slightly cloudy fluid through the urethra. That fluid is made up of water, a bit of urea, creatinine, and a magical compound called prostatic-specific antigen (PSA)—which comes from the Skene's glands, also known as the female prostate. In other words, it's real. It's not just pee.

And here's the thing: Not all women squirt**.** Not all want to. And that's okay. It's not a sign of sexual success or failure. It's just one flavor of release, one form of expression. Some women can squirt with internal pressure, some with clit + G-spot combo, some during intense orgasms, and some not at all.

What matters more is: Are you *feeling* it? Are you present? Are you turned on and tuned into what your body is asking for? If the answer is yes, then whether you soak a towel or just melt into the sheets, it's perfect.

The Pleasure Behind You

Welcome to the conversation on anal pleasure. Now let's clear this up: there isn't technically a second G-spot tucked away back there. But—and this is a very sexy "but"—what you *can* find is a deep, rich pleasure that feels very G-spot adjacent.

Here's why:
The rectum and the vaginal wall are right next door neighbors. That backdoor stimulation? It can indirectly put pressure on your G-spot, A-spot, and all kinds of internal nerve endings that light up like a pinball machine. Add in the pudendal nerve, which carries pleasure signals from the clit, vagina, and anus all at once? It's giving full-body vibrational bliss.

Now, let's not romanticize this without keeping it real:

- Lube is law. The anus doesn't self-lubricate. No exceptions.

- Go slow. This is not the time for jackhammer energy. Think "respectful explorer," not "reckless pirate."

- Relaxation is key. If your body says no, listen. If your brain won't shut up, take your time. Tension is the enemy of pleasure back there.

- Gently bear down—push like you're about to poop—to help your muscles relax and open comfortably.

- Cleanliness, communication, and consent are non-negotiables.
- Positions like spooning or doggy-style (with *gentle entry!*) often help you relax and allow you to control the depth and angle. You're the conductor here, not just a passenger.

For some women, anal play feels… *meh*. For others? It's orgasmic, especially when combined with clitoral or vaginal stimulation. Either way, it's not about being wild or freaky for someone else. It's about exploring your body with your permission, your curiosity, and your rules. There is power in owning all parts of your pleasure. Even the parts behind you.

So, if you ever feel the call to explore, know this: there's no shame in seeking pleasure where others told you it didn't belong. Your body, your map, your orgasm.

Rewiring the Erotic Mind

Reclaiming Sensuality for You

That turned-on feeling? That heat in your belly, that ache between your thighs, that magnetic pull toward sensation? It's not just about sex. That's life force. That's you lit up from the inside. Sexual energy is the root of your creativity, your confidence, your power to manifest. It's the same energy that births babies, books, businesses, and breakthroughs. It doesn't need a partner, a vibrator, or even an orgasm to matter. It's your essence. That shiver you feel when you're deeply inspired? That's her. That rush of boldness when you say something without filtering it first? Her. The sudden burst of clarity that hits you mid-shower? Yep, still her.
You don't have to use it sexually for it to feed you. Reclaiming pleasure in your everyday life—not just orgasm, but ordinary sensuality—unlocks something ancient.

You start catching your reflection and winking instead of criticizing. You touch your neck mid-lotion and pause because damn, that felt good. You go for a walk and feel your hips sway like poetry. You speak with more certainty. You glow with less makeup. You start walking like your thighs were hand-carved by the divine.

Pleasure isn't a distraction from your purpose. It's a direct line to it. It opens the channel between your root and your crown, between your desire and your destiny. If you've ever had your best ideas after an orgasm, this is why. Turned-on women are powerful. Not because of what they do, but because of who they remember they are.

The lingerie is cute. The flirtation is fun. The selfies hit harder when the light is just right. But deep down, this reclamation isn't for attention. It's not for the 'gram. It's not for the male gaze. It's not for the ex you hope is watching your glow-up. It's for you.

To feel connected. To feel present. To feel powerful in your skin without needing to perform or be perfect. Sensuality isn't how you look. It's how you feel. It's how you sip your tea. It's how you dance when no one's watching. It's how you say "mmm" when something tastes good. And when you reclaim it for yourself, everyone else just gets lucky to witness the aftermath.

1. Start with your senses
Sensuality is sensory. Begin with one sense at a time and build rituals around them.

- **Touch:** Wear soft clothes. Sleep naked. Layer on oils, not just lotion. Rub your shoulders and say, *damn, I feel good today.*

- **Smell:** Light candles that smell like seduction. Use body washes that make you close your eyes in the shower. Let scent become your signature.

- **Sound:** Create a playlist that makes your hips move without permission. Play it when you clean, cook, or do nothing at all.

- **Taste:** Eat slowly. Savor your food. Lick the spoon like it flirted with you.

- **Sight:** Curate your space. Mood lighting. Velvet pillows. Maybe a full body mirror that says *you're the moment*. Because you are.

2. Romanticize the hell out of your routines
Make brushing your hair an act of worship. Make your skincare routine feel like a spa day. Pour your coffee like you're in a 90s R&B video. Slow down and notice what makes you feel delicious.

3. Move like you're the main character
Dance in the mirror. Take long walks with extra hip. Twerk in the kitchen while the water boils. Movement isn't just about exercise, it's about expression.
Let your body lead. Let her loosen. Let her remember that she's meant to move with rhythm, not rigidity.

4. Create a sensual night ritual
Not for productivity. Not for performance. For *pleasure*.

- Body oiling. Even a sprits of a light perfume before bed can set a tone of self admiration
- Breathwork or mirror affirmations

- A robe that makes you feel like a wealthy widow with secrets
- Journaling to reconnect with your body's voice
End your night with softness. Not screens. Not stress.

Sensuality isn't how you pose. It's how you exist.
It's a tone you carry. And when you claim that without needing applause, the world notices anyway. People can't name it, but they feel it. The softness. The strength. The magnetism of a woman who turned herself on and didn't ask for permission.

Intimacy with Yourself

Let's stop calling it "just masturbating" like it's a quick shame-rush in the dark. Touch your body like she's art, not a problem to be fixed. Don't rush to the finish line. Explore. Listen. Be curious. Touch yourself like you're simmering in self-worth. Let it be slow. Let it be messy. Let it be ugly-crying if it needs to be. That's healing. If you laugh? That's release. If you moan like it's your own rebirth? That's power.

Your orgasm doesn't need to be perfect.
It just needs to be yours. And if it brings release, clarity, creativity, or joy—know that you just performed a ritual more powerful than most people ever allow themselves to experience.

Cycle-Based Sex Drive

If you've ever felt wildly turned on one week, then completely unbothered the next, you're not flaky, you're just cyclical. Your libido is tied to your hormone cycle. Once you start working with it instead of against it—whole new world.

Follicular phase (after your period):
Estrogen is rising, and so is your mood. You're playful, energized, and maybe a little extra flirty in texts without even realizing it. This is a great time to try new positions, lingerie, or even suggest a date night where you set the tone.

Ovulation (mid-cycle):
You're magnetic. Your skin glows. Your body wants connection. Your libido is at its peak, and your scent, energy, and confidence are all turned up. This is the time to explore what makes you feel powerful. Toys, dirty talk, mirrors, lace, whatever speaks to your primal self.

Luteal phase (before your period):
Your body slows down and tunes in. You might crave intimacy that's deep and slow. You might also want space, quiet, or to cry after a back rub. All of it is valid. Ask yourself: do I need pleasure or do I need peace? Sometimes the answer is both.

Menstrual phase (your period):
You might think you're least likely to be turned on, but don't be surprised if blood flow increases sensitivity and makes orgasm

feel even more intense. If you're comfortable, this can be a powerful time to connect with yourself or your partner. Soft sheets, towels, and open communication can turn this phase into something sacred instead of shameful.

There is no wrong time to feel desire. There is only your time. Tune in. Trust it. Let your cycle be your compass, not your cage.

Enhancing Pleasure

Sex Toys

Let's get one thing straight: toys aren't cheating.
They're not just for when you're single or when your partner "isn't doing it right." They're extensions of your pleasure. They're amplifiers.

Want a buzz that builds? Try a bullet.
Want air pulses that literally mimic oral? Rose.
Want internal pressure and clit vibes? Look into rabbit-style vibrators (the dual-threat queens).
Want to explore depth, stretch, or fullness? Glass, silicone, or weighted wands are your go-to.
And if you want your whole body in on the action? Wand massagers. You don't need a drawer full (but no judgment if you do). You just need permission. To explore. To experiment. To find out what makes your body light up like a damn galaxy.

Learn yourself first, babe. If you can't please yourself, how the hell you gonna let someone else do it? (Can I get an amen?)

Your body isn't a puzzle for someone else to solve. She's a sacred language for you to learn.
What feels good? Where do you like to be touched?
Do you like soft and slow, or deep and rhythmic?
Do you need music? Scents? Movement? Affirmations? A toy? Silence? Learning yourself isn't just sexual—it's spiritual. It's reclaiming territory that was never meant to be colonized by shame, silence, or someone else's preferences. Self-pleasure is a form of prayer. And your orgasm is a response.

Now this next part is for the women in the back hiding their bullet in a sock drawer like it's contraband. If your partner can't handle your pleasure, that's their insecurity, not your problem. If your partner shames you for using toys, exploring your body, or knowing what you like… that's a red flag, not a personality trait. If they're threatened by your pleasure, that says more about their insecurity than your desire. You shouldn't have to hide your vibrator like it's something to be embarrassed about. You shouldn't feel guilty for knowing yourself and taking care of your own needs. If anything, toys can be part of your intimacy together if you're comfortable. Bring them in. Let them be part of the moment, not separate from it. Let your partner watch. Let them use it on you. Let them learn what turns you on instead of guessing. Because the truth is, a partner who wants you to feel good will *never* be offended by what helps you get there.

When you know your body, you become unshakable in the bedroom. Once you know what you like... the next step is sharing it. Out loud. With intention. With audacity.

Let Them Know What You Like

Your partner isn't a mind reader and your pleasure isn't a puzzle they get extra credit for solving on their own. If you want to be touched a certain way, say it. If they're going too fast, slow them down. You are not here to perform while hoping they eventually stumble on the right spot.

This isn't about being bossy. It's about being *in tune* with your body and generous enough to share the directions. You shouldn't have to hold your breath and hope they figure it out. You shouldn't have to fake it just to protect their ego. And you shouldn't be afraid of making a request—especially when your body is on the line. You're not "too much" for needing more. You're not "difficult" because your pleasure requires intention.

You're not "demanding" because you want connection, rhythm, communication, or foreplay that actually involves your entire body.

You are allowed to say:

"Slower."
"Right there."
"Softer."
"Use your tongue."
"Let's use the toy."
"Harder."
"I need a break."
"Keep going."
"Try this instead."
"I don't like that."

You're allowed to ask for it without overexplaining. You're allowed to guide without apologizing. You're allowed to moan instructions if you want to… or whisper them, or write them down, or say them before sex even begins. And if someone reacts with defensiveness, shame, or offense instead of curiosity, maturity, and desire to learn? That's not a lover, that's a liability. The right partner doesn't take offense when you speak up, they lean in. They want to know what makes you melt. They want to be part of your pleasure, not the reason you go quiet in your own body. The right partner asks what you like, pays attention when you answer, and adjusts with pride, not poutiness.

Remember, you're not there to be quiet and accommodating. You're not there to "make them feel like they're good at sex" while you're left unsatisfied and disconnected. You're there to

be *in it*. To be present, to be met, to be touched the way you actually want to be
touched. And if that makes you feel exposed? Vulnerable? Nervous the first few times? That's okay. It's not about always being bold, it's about being brave enough to choose yourself. When you speak up, you don't just invite better sex. You invite real intimacy. And babe… that's the whole point.

Common Kinks & Pleasures to Explore

Do you like to be praised, adored, and asked if you're a good girl? Or do you crave control, power, and having someone on their knees for you? Do you melt with tenderness or crave a little roughness? A soft grip on your waist, or a playful hand around your throat? Wax on your thighs or velvet around your wrists?

Yeah. Let's talk about *that*.

(If you're curious, you're already halfway there.)

- **Sensory Play:** blindfolds, silk scarves, feathers, ice, warm oils

- **Impact Play:** spanking, light slapping, flogging (consensual + controlled)

- **Power Exchange:** dominance & submission (D/s), being "in control" or surrendering fully

- **Praise Kink:** being called "good girl," adored, worshipped

- **Degradation Kink:** being called names, rough talk (ONLY when mutually consensual)

- **Wax Play:** warm candle wax dripped on skin – use body-safe candles only

- **Bondage:** handcuffs, ropes, under-bed restraints, Velcro ties

- **Roleplay:** fantasy fulfillment – nurse, goddess, stranger, boss

- **Breath Play:** controlled pressure around the neck (advanced, must be safe, consensual)

- **Exhibitionism:** being watched

- **Voyeurism:** watching someone else

This isn't about doing all the things. It's about giving yourself permission to explore what makes you feel powerful, desired, free, soft, wild, or surrendered. You can be a pillow princess one night and a dom the next. You can whisper, command, giggle, or growl. Whatever it is, own it. Communicate it. Enjoy it. You are allowed to ask for what you want. You are allowed to guide the moment. And you are allowed to say "harder," "slower," "yes," or "absolutely not."

Whew. Okay. Let's take a breath, maybe sip some water, and cool things down. While kinks, toys, and positions are fun (and necessary), they're only part of the story. Behind every surge of desire, every dry spell, every "I'm ready to climb him like a tree" moment and every "don't even touch me" phase—there's a quiet crew running the show… your hormones. Our MVP's are back. Let's get into how they play a role in your sex life.

Hormones & Libido

Your sex drive isn't just about "being in the mood", it's a whole-body experience that relies on hormonal balance, blood flow, stress levels, and even gut health.

The Big Players in Libido

Testosterone
This hormone fuels desire, sensitivity, and pleasure. If it's too low, your libido takes a nosedive.

Estrogen
Keeps vaginal tissues hydrated and sensitive. Low estrogen = dryness, discomfort, and *why does this feel different?*

Progesterone
The relaxing hormone. If it's too low, you feel anxious, wired, and definitely not in the mood.

Cortisol
High stress kills your libido faster than bad Wi-Fi. If you're constantly in fight-or-flight mode, your body prioritizes survival over sex.

Dopamine & Oxytocin
These are the pleasure and bonding chemicals that make intimacy exciting and fulfilling. If you're not getting enough dopamine (from joy, pleasure, and fun), your sex drive suffers.

Signs Your Hormones Are Killing Your Libido:

- You're never in the mood, no matter how much you love your partner.

- Sex feels like a chore, not something enjoyable.

- Vaginal dryness or discomfort during intimacy (low estrogen alert!).

- You feel exhausted, moody, or disconnected.

- You crave sugar, carbs, or caffeine more than physical touch.

- High stress, anxiety, or burnout is taking over.

The good news? You can reset your hormones and bring your libido back to life. Let's talk about how.

Natural Libido Boosters

Start with what you're eating. Certain foods naturally support hormone balance, blood flow, and arousal.

Dark Chocolate
Boosts dopamine and serotonin (*aka: puts you in a good mood*).

Avocados
Packed with B vitamins, which support sex hormone production.

Berries
High in antioxidants, which improve blood flow to your lady parts.

Maca Root
The ultimate hormone-balancing superfood for increased libido, energy, and mood.

Protein
Supports testosterone production, which fuels desire.

A Glass of Red Wine
Contains resveratrol, a natural blood flow booster (but don't overdo it—too much alcohol numbs sensation).

Pumpkin Seeds & Brazil Nuts
High in zinc and selenium, which support testosterone levels and orgasmic function.

Medications & Libido

Certain medications—including hormonal birth control, SSRIs, antihistamines, and even some blood pressure meds—can mess with your libido, vaginal moisture, or mood. It's not always talked about, but it should be. If you've been feeling "off," don't assume it's just in your head. Talk to a provider who actually listens, and track what changed when you started your meds. You deserve answers, not assumptions.

The Big Stress-Sex Connection

If your brain won't shut off, neither will your body. Stress is the biggest libido killer. It raises cortisol, which lowers testosterone, blocks dopamine, and dries up desire like the Sahara.

Magnesium
Helps relax your muscles, reduce anxiety, and improve sleep (*which = more energy for fun things*).

Massage & Sensory Play
Touch boosts oxytocin and dopamine, making you feel closer, calmer, and more connected.

Music, Candles, & Mood Lighting
Set the mood. Your brain needs cues to shift from stress mode to pleasure mode.

Prioritize Sleep
Sleep deprivation turns into low libido, low energy, and hormonal chaos.

The Hormonal Benefits of Getting Yours

Orgasms aren't just fun, they're actually amazing for your hormones, mood, and stress levels. They:

- **Lower Cortisol** - Helps relieve stress, anxiety, and tension.

- **Boosts Estrogen & Progesterone** - Keeps vaginal tissues healthy and hormones balanced.

- **Increases Blood Flow** - Helps with sensitivity, pleasure, and natural lubrication.

- **Raises Oxytocin (The Bonding Hormone)** - Makes you feel happier, more connected, and emotionally fulfilled.

Moral of the story? Prioritize pleasure. Your hormones will thank you. With that in mind, pleasure should *never* come at someone else's expense. What balances one body should never break another.

When Pleasure Wasn't Safe

Let's pause for the women who've been harmed under the name of pleasure. Maybe you've had a partner who treated sex like a need you were supposed to fulfill and not a connection you get to choose.
Maybe you've been with someone who got moody, cold, or even cruel if they didn't get what they wanted.
Maybe you were taught that their pleasure mattered more than your comfort. Or that if you said no, you'd pay for it in silence or tension for the rest of the day.
If that's been your experience, it makes sense if the word *pleasure* feels loaded. If it doesn't sound soft or healing. If it sounds like pressure, performance, or punishment. That is real. And it deserves to be named.

This chapter is about reclaiming what was always yours, the kind of pleasure that comes from listening to your body, not abandoning it. The kind of pleasure that heals, not harms. You are not here to regulate someone else's cortisol by sacrificing your own peace. You are not here to be available just so someone else can be emotionally stable. That's not intimacy. That's obligation. And you deserve so much more than that.

When I say *prioritize pleasure*, I don't mean serve it up on command. I mean find the kind that replenishes you. That nourishes your nervous system. That quiets the shame, the fear, the inner freeze. That makes you feel more like yourself when it's over, not less. You don't owe anyone access to your body in order to keep the peace.

Let this be your new standard:
Pleasure that feels safe.
Pleasure that's mutual.
Pleasure that honors *you*, too.

Before we end this chapter, I want to speak to the women reading who haven't always felt safe in their own bodies. Who've had their pleasure taken instead of invited. Who've said "no" in ways that were ignored.
Who've stayed silent because they froze. Who've had partners they trusted push past boundaries because "you didn't say stop," or "you're mine," or "you owe me."

Maybe you weren't held down. Maybe you didn't scream. Maybe you told yourself it wasn't *that* bad. But something inside you disconnected, and you've been carrying the silence ever since.

I see you.

You're not dramatic. You're not confused. You're not "making it up." You were violated.
Even if they never called it that.
Even if you went along with it.
Even if you loved them.
Even if it didn't "look like rape."
It was still wrong. And it left something behind.

I've been there, too. I know what it feels like to have someone or a partner press themselves into your body when your spirit has already left the room. To be touched with entitlement instead of care. To go quiet because fighting back feels harder than just getting it over with. I know what it does to your sense of safety. Your sexuality. Your softness. Your power. And I know how hard it is to try to reclaim pleasure after that.

This chapter wasn't written to bypass your pain. It wasn't written with false light and glittery sex tips. It was written *for* you. For every woman who is learning how to trust her body again. For every woman who wants to feel something good without flinching. For every woman who has decided that her story doesn't end with what was taken from her.

You are more than what they did.
You are more than the moments you endured.
You are not dirty.
You are not broken.
You are not less of a woman because someone treated your body like a thing.

I won't pretend this work is easy. Reclaiming pleasure after pain is slow, layered, and sacred. But you are worthy of every step. You are allowed to go at your own pace. You are allowed to take breaks. To cry in the middle of touching yourself. To stop mid-sex and say, "actually, no." To not want to be touched at all. Or to finally say, "yes," and mean it fully.

My heart breaks for how many of us have been harmed by people who were supposed to love us. And still, I believe in our healing. I believe in your return to yourself. In your softness. In your rage. In your right to feel joy in your body again. Not because someone gives it to you, but because you *choose* it.

This world has not always been kind to women. Especially not when it comes to pleasure. But let this be the turning point. Let this be the page where you remember:
You're allowed to want.
You're allowed to feel.
You're allowed to heal.
And none of it will ever be too much.
You are the author of your body now.
And this chapter belongs to you.

Feminine Upgrades

Your pelvic floor muscles play a HUGE role in sexual pleasure. A strong pelvic floor equals better orgasms, better blood flow, and better sensation. A weak or too-tight pelvic floor can lead to low sensation, discomfort, and even urinary leaks (*which is NOT the kind of excitement we're looking for*).

Signs Your Pelvic Floor Needs Some Love:

- Low sensation or difficulty climaxing (*yup, that's pelvic floor-related*).

- Pain or tightness during intimacy.

- Leaking when you sneeze, cough, or laugh (*if you know, you know*).

- Lower back pain or hip tension (*your pelvic floor muscles connect to these areas!*).

What Helps

Kegels
Contract and hold for 3-5 seconds, then release. Do 10-15 reps a day (*but don't overdo it – too much tightening can actually make things worse!*).

Pelvic Floor Relaxation

If your pelvic floor is too tight, you need to stretch and relax it (*try deep breathing, hip openers, or even working with a pelvic floor therapist*).

Consistent Movement

Walking, squats, and yoga improve blood flow to the pelvis, which boosts sensation and lubrication.

Enhancing Your Nectar

Your body is sacred chemistry. What you eat, how you move, and even how you feel can influence the moisture, scent, and taste of your feminine essence. Here are natural ways to enhance the flavor of your honey pot.

Pineapple Juice & Sweet Fruits

There's a reason pineapple has earned a reputation in the bedroom. High in natural sugars and enzymes like bromelain, pineapple may help make vaginal secretions sweeter and more appealing in taste. Anecdotal evidence supports this, especially when combined with a clean, plant-rich diet. Other helpful fruits include:

- Mango
- Papaya
- Watermelon

- Apples
- Kiwi

Pair them with good hydration for full effect.

Okra Water
Okra contains mucilage—a natural, slippery substance that supports internal lubrication. While formal research is limited, traditional medicine praises okra water for its ability to increase cervical fluid and vaginal wetness. Many women in TTC (trying to conceive) and holistic womb health circles swear by it. Okra is also rich in folate, magnesium, and vitamin C. Great for reproductive vitality.

To try it, slice 3-5 okra pods, soak overnight in 1-2 cups of water, and drink the mucilage-infused water the next morning.

Fenugreek Seeds
Fenugreek can subtly sweeten body odor and secretions when taken consistently. Its phytoestrogens also support natural lubrication by mimicking estrogen. You can take it in capsule form or steep the seeds to make a slightly bitter tea.

Fenugreek may affect blood sugar and hormones. Avoid during pregnancy unless advised.

Chlorophyll Drops, Parsley, and Mint
These internal deodorizers help purify from the inside out. Try chlorophyll drops in water, green smoothies with parsley or mint, or herbal teas like peppermint and spearmint.

Aloe Vera Juice (Inner Fillet Only)
Aloe vera's soothing and lubricating properties may help increase natural wetness and balance vaginal pH. Make sure to use organic, decolorized aloe vera juice (inner fillet only) to avoid laxative effects.

Flaxseed & Omega-3s
Healthy fats improve tissue softness, stretch, and wetness. Include flaxseed, chia, walnuts, avocado, evening primrose oil, or omega-3 supplements in your routine.

Herbs for Sweetness & Wetness
Teas or tinctures with damiana, shatavari, red raspberry leaf, or licorice root (in moderation) can support natural lubrication and hormonal balance.

Erotic Movement & Sensual Touch
Dancing, yoga, twerking, stretching, or even massaging oil into your body can stimulate arousal energetically – not just physically. Turn yourself on with yourself. Wetness often begins in the mind and builds from there.

Mutual Flavor, Mutual Care
(A subtle little fruit-forward finesse for the fellas)

Let's talk about *his* flavor for a second. If your partner is a male and things are getting mouthy in the bedroom, just know: what he eats shows up on the menu, too.

His diet directly affects how he tastes, and if you've ever paused mid-oral wondering why it's giving battery acid and protein shake, you are not alone.

Sweet, water-rich fruits like pineapple, kiwi, mango, strawberries, and watermelon can help naturally balance and sweeten the flavor of semen over time. The same goes for staying hydrated and cutting back on acidic or pungent foods like red meat, onions, garlic, and too much caffeine or alcohol.

If he's constantly downing energy drinks and skipping greens, it *will* show up in the vibe... and the taste.

So, be playful about it. Drop a smoothie in his hand. Pack a fruit bowl next to his sandwich. Casually offer him water like you're *not* on a mission.

And if he starts acting picky about the health push? Just remind him – If he wants you to go down, he better not taste like a pharmacy aisle. Tell him: "No one wants to taste regret, bro. Grab a pineapple." If he wants you to treat it like a snack, he better not taste like a struggle. Because oral goes both ways, babe. Mutual pleasure means mutual care. When both of you are feeding your bodies like sacred temples, the chemistry hits different. Taste becomes part of the experience, not something you try to ignore… and you both deserve that.

When to Seek Professional Help

If you've done the inner work, explored the tools in this chapter, and still feel disconnected from your body or pleasure, it may be time to reach out for support. Whether you're dealing with a low sex drive, painful intimacy, or emotional shutdowns around sex, you deserve care. You don't have to carry it alone.

Emotional & Psychological Concerns

- A persistent lack of desire that doesn't shift, no matter what you've tried

- Anxiety, fear, or discomfort around touch or intimacy

- Trauma from past sexual harm, coercion, or emotional neglect

- Depression or anxiety that makes it hard to feel aroused or emotionally present

- Body image struggles or low self-worth that interfere with connection

- Relationship breakdowns, emotional distance, or unresolved tension

- Postpartum depression or identity changes that make you feel disconnected from your sensuality

Physical & Medical Issues

- Pain during sex, including vaginal, vulvar, or pelvic pain
- Vaginismus (tightness or muscle clenching that makes penetration difficult or painful)

- Anorgasmia (difficulty or inability to reach orgasm)

- Hormonal imbalances like low estrogen, low testosterone, or thyroid dysfunction

- Pelvic floor dysfunction (tightness, weakness, or lack of coordination)

- Recurring infections like BV, yeast infections, or UTIs that affect intimacy

- Menopause-related shifts like dryness, thinning tissue, or reduced sensitivity

- Side effects from medications (especially antidepressants, hormonal birth control, or SSRIs)

When to Reach Out

You deserve support if:

- Sex feels more like pressure than connection

- You feel emotionally or physically numb during intimacy

- You've lost your sense of sensuality and don't know how to get it back

- You feel stuck in shame or fear when it comes to your own pleasure

- You're healing from trauma and ready to feel safe in your body again

Professionals Who Can Help

- Pelvic floor physical therapists
- Trauma-informed or sex-positive therapists
- Somatic sex educators or holistic intimacy coaches
- OB/GYN or women's health providers
- Endocrinologists (for hormone-related concerns)
- Mental health professionals who understand sexual trauma, anxiety, or depression

Okay… can we just take a moment to breathe and acknowledge the fact that you just made it through this chapter? A quarter of the entire book. And every single word deserved to be here.

Low libido isn't just a phase, a punishment, or a side effect of being "too busy" or "too broken." It's your body waving a flag—asking you to come back home. Your sensual self isn't gone… she's just been buried under burnout, hormone chaos, unhealed wounds, and stories that never belonged to you in the first place.

You are not too much. You are not "behind." You are not broken. You are a rhythmic, radiant, ever-evolving force.

So whether you're melting into solo sessions, reconnecting with a partner, healing after pain, or just figuring out what turns you on again, honor the process. Let pleasure be your compass. Let your orgasm be your affirmation. And if something's off? Seek the support you deserve. Because the truth is: your sensuality isn't optional.

It's sacred.
It's healing.
It's yours.

So light the candle.
Touch with intention.

Ask for what you want.

And the next time your body opens, softens, or pulses with pleasure – receive it. Because that, babe, is your birthright. You're allowed to feel good again. You're allowed to take your time. And you're allowed to want more.

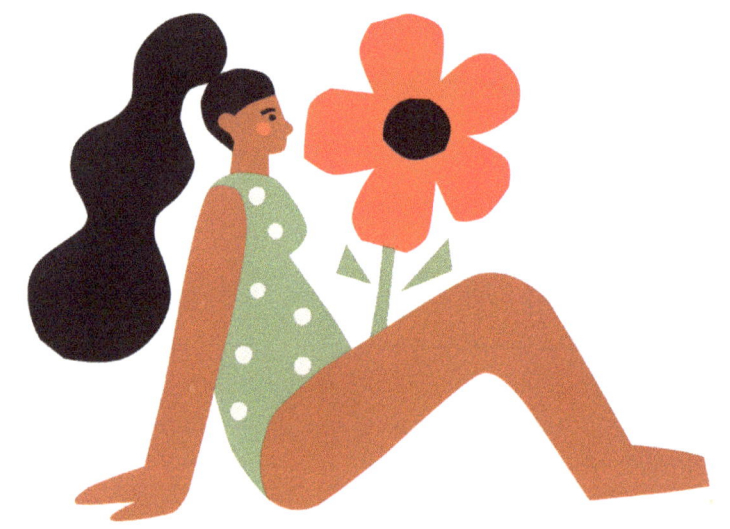

Chapter 6
WOMB SERVICE

Whether you're baby-crazy, baby-curious, or proudly on Team No Kids Ever, understanding fertility is key to owning your reproductive health. Your cycle isn't just about making babies. It's basically your body's monthly report card. So, let's decode those hormonal messages.

Birth Control Breakdown

Let's get one thing straight: you don't owe anyone a baby. Not society, not your mama, not your partner—not even your own uterus on the days she feels extra emotional. Birth control isn't just a backup plan, it's a tool of self-governance. A boundary. A whole power move. We're starting here because reproductive freedom is step one in womb wellness. And knowing how your birth control works (or doesn't) is just as important as knowing why you're using it. So before we talk about ovulation, cervical mucus, or any of that baby-making magic, let's talk options. Let's talk side effects. Let's talk hormones. Let's talk control—and how to take it back.

Hormonal birth control isn't the enemy, it's a tool. But every tool comes with trade-offs.

- **The Pill**: Prevents ovulation, lightens periods, can stabilize acne, but may lower libido or cause mood shifts.

- **The Patch**: Delivers steady hormones through the skin. Convenient, but similar side effects to the pill.

- **IUD (Hormonal)**: Thins uterine lining and thickens cervical mucus. Low-maintenance, but can alter bleeding patterns.

- **Copper IUD**: Hormone-free. Prevents pregnancy by creating a sperm-hostile environment. Heavier periods are common.
- **Implants & Shots**: Long-term options that can affect mood, weight, and cycle regularity
- Listen to your body. If something feels off, you're allowed to explore alternatives.

Breaking Up With Birth Control

If you're ditching hormonal birth control, here's how to transition smoothly (and avoid feeling like a hormonal mess).

Nutritional TLC

- Liver-loving herbs like milk thistle, turmeric, burdock, and dandelion root will be your detox squad.

- Hormone helpers: Vitex (chaste tree berry) gives your progesterone a pep talk.

Lifestyle Upgrades

- Chill vibes only. Yoga, meditation, or aggressively lighting candles—pick your calming activity.

- Move your body—but don't stress it out.

Track Your Cycle

- Use an app or journal. Your cycle is your monthly blueprint—listen carefully.

- If things stay weird, check with your doc. Sometimes your body needs backup.

Hormone Free Birth Control

For those dodging pregnancy without the pill, lets channel your inner fertility detective.

Fertility Awareness Methods (FAMs)

Basal Body Temperature (BBT)
Take your temp first thing in the morning, every single day (yep, like a fertility-obsessed scientist). Look for a noticeable rise—about 0.5° to 1°F after ovulation. If it stays elevated for 18+ days, surprise—you might be pregnant.

Cervical Mucus
Yes, checking your discharge is a thing. Gross? Maybe. But useful.
- Fertile mucus: Slippery, stretchy, clear - like raw egg whites. This is prime baby-making mucus.
- Non-fertile mucus: Sticky, creamy, dry. Sperm-blocking mucus, basically your body's natural "not today" signal.

- Track changes daily. When you notice the slippery, stretchy phase, that's go-time for conception (or caution time for avoiding pregnancy).

Symptothermal Method
Combine the above for maximum baby making or baby-dodging accuracy. Done perfectly? 99%. Done lazily? More like 76%. Be consistent or prepare for surprises.

Calendar-Based Methods

Standard Days Method**:** Only for the lucky ones with clockwork cycles.

Rhythm Method**:** Kinda works, but if your cycle is unpredictable, consider this *Living like Larry (on the edge)*.

Ovulation

Ovulation isn't just about getting pregnant, it's your body's way of saying, "*Hey girl, we good?*". If your cycle is regular with clear ovulation signs? Chef's kiss Period going rogue or ghosting you entirely? That's a red flag waving high and clear. Tracking your cycle isn't just for those trying to get knocked up.

What Even is Ovulation?

It's the main event of your cycle. Each month (in theory), one of your ovaries releases an egg. That egg floats down the fallopian tube like she's waiting for a date (sperm) to show up. If sperm arrives? Fertilization might happen. If not? The egg dissolves, and your body prepares to shed the uterine lining— aka, your period. In short: ovulation is your body saying, *"Just in case you want a baby, I'm ready."*

But even if you're not trying to conceive, ovulation still matters. Why? Because it's a sign your hormones are flowing, your stress isn't hijacking your system, and your reproductive organs are functioning like the divine machinery they are. When you're ovulating regularly, it means your body is in sync. And when you're not? It could be your first whisper that something's out of alignment—whether it's stress, under-eating, overtraining, PCOS, or just life doing too much.

Fertility

Wanting to get pregnant is tender, powerful, and sometimes a little scary. There's hope. There's pressure. There's a hundred questions you don't know how to ask yet. And that's okay. Because this next is not just about sperm-meets-egg. It's about building a strong, supported foundation before the baby bump. It's about understanding how your cycle works, how to time things right, and how to give your body the nourishment, rest, and love it needs to prepare for new life.

Whether you're ready to start trying this month or just beginning to daydream, consider this your gentle guide into conscious conception—rooted in knowledge, grace, and a whole lot of self-trust.

Busting Fertility Myths

Myth: Stopping birth control wrecks your fertility forever.
Reality: Your ovaries don't hold grudges. Most people bounce back just fine.
Myth: Women's fertility nose-dives off a cliff at 35.
Reality: While fertility does decline with age, it's more of a gentle slide than a dramatic drop-off. Chill.

Myth: Men stay fertile *forever*.
Reality: Sorry fellas, but sperm quality also takes a hit with age. No one's immune to Father Time.

Fertility Boosters

Whether you're baby-making or just balancing your hormones, here's how to keep your reproductive health thriving.

`Nutrition: Fertility Fuel

- Eat the rainbow (and no, I don't mean Skittles). Load up on fresh produce, lean proteins, and healthy fats.

- Antioxidants, baby. Berries, nuts, and leafy greens = MVPs for sperm and egg quality.

Stress Management

- Zen out however you prefer – Yoga, meditation, or deep breathing – pick your poison and relax.

- Prioritize Sleep. Aim for 7-8 hours unless you enjoy looking and feeling like a zombie.

Move It (But Don't Overdo It)

- Regular movement like walking, swimming, or dancing like nobody's watching gets that blood flowing and hormones balanced.

- Avoid overdoing it. Fertility doesn't vibe with exhaustion. Balance, babe.

The Emotional Side of Fertility

No one tells you that trying to conceive (or trying *not* to) can stir up everything from hope and heartbreak to rage and radical surrender. Fertility isn't just physical. It's emotional, spiritual, and deeply personal.

Some months, your body might feel like it's betraying you. Other months, you're holding onto hope like it's your last lifeline. Whether you're navigating miscarriage, infertility, or simply feeling disconnected from your womb, please know: you are not broken. You are not late. You are not less than.

This chapter isn't just about tips and timelines. It's about honoring the tender, often invisible journey of being a woman in a body that was never meant to run on shame or silence.

A Two-Player Game

Fertility is a duet, not a solo act. Society loves to pin baby-making struggles on women, but the truth? Infertility issues are split 50/50 between partners. So if there's a bump in the reproductive road, both players need to get checked out. Teamwork makes the dream work.

It's not just the egg that makes the magic happen —sperm has a VIP role, too. A father's health and lifestyle before conception can impact pregnancy outcomes more than most people realize.

Dad's Placenta Role

Did you know that paternal genes help build the placenta? One gene, PEG10, is basically dad's way of making sure the baby gets all the nutrients it needs. If that gene isn't working, pregnancy can get complicated quickly.

Dad Lifestyle Checks

- Smoking? Bad for sperm and baby's birth weight.

- Toxic jobs? Watch out for fertility and pregnancy health.
- Older dads? Sperm quality dips with age, raising genetic mutation risks.

Genetic Screening & Future Planning

If fertility runs deep in your thoughts or if your family history includes ovarian, uterine, or breast cancer, it might be time to think beyond ovulation strips and BBT charts. Ask your doctor about genetic screening, especially if you're considering pregnancy later in life. Tests like BRCA1/2 can give insight into your reproductive risks and options for proactive care.
This isn't fear-mongering, it's power. Knowing what's written in your genes doesn't define you. But it can guide you.

Prenatals: Not Just for Pregnancy

Prenatal vitamins aren't just for pregnancy. You should be taking them before conception (to build nutrient reserves) and after birth (especially if breastfeeding). They support:

- Folate for neural tube development
- Iron for blood supply
- DHA for baby's brain
- And YOU–for energy, healing, and hormone balance

Postpartum & Hormonal Recovery

Postpartum doesn't come with a guidebook or a finish line. You're healing, bleeding, barely sleeping, maybe nursing, and trying to remember who you are underneath the spit-up and stretchy mesh panties. It's raw. It's real. And for a lot of women, it's heavy.

The baby blues are common in those first couple weeks. Random crying spells, mood swings, irritability, feeling overwhelmed or like you're on the edge of something but don't know what. But when it lingers… when it gets deeper… that's when we step into postpartum depression, and it's not just "a little sad." It can feel like disconnection. Numbness. Rage. Emptiness. Guilt. Loneliness. And no, it doesn't mean you're failing. It means your hormones are recalibrating. Your nervous system is stretched thin. And your body is asking for support.

Ways to Support Your Mood

These won't fix everything, but they can help you feel like you again, little by little.

Get Sunlight
Try to get outside, even if it's just for 10-20 minutes. Sunlight helps regulate melatonin, increase serotonin, and improve your

circadian rhythm—all crucial for mood and hormone recovery. No sunshine? Use a light therapy lamp. Yes, it's that serious.

Grounding Meals

Skip the cold smoothies for now. Focus on foods that feel like comfort and nourishment:
- Broths, soups, and stews
- Cooked veggies
- Healthy fats like avocado or olive oil
- Iron-rich foods like spinach, beets, dates

Your body just created life… it's okay to feed it like royalty.

Supportive Supplements

Talk to your provider first, but common postpartum supports include:

- Omega-3s (especially DHA) for mood
- Vitamin D (low levels = low energy)
- Magnesium for sleep and nervous system recovery
- B vitamins to replenish what pregnancy and breastfeeding burned through

Touch & Connection

Skin-to-skin with baby. Hugs from your partner. A hand massage. Anything that reminds your body it's safe to relax. Physical affection releases oxytocin, the hormone of bonding and calm.

Expression & Emotional Unpacking
You don't have to journal every day or write a memoir, but carving out even five minutes to brain-dump your feelings—the rage, the grief, the joy, the fear—gives those emotions somewhere to land that *isn't your chest*

Lower the Bar
Some days, getting dressed is the victory. Let that be enough. The laundry can wait. The dishes can sit. You are recovering, not performing.

And If It's More Than You Can Carry…
If the fog won't lift, if you don't feel like yourself at all, or if you feel numb instead of connected Talk to someone. A therapist. A postpartum doula. A doctor. Your favorite auntie. Anyone who won't gaslight your pain or hand you a Bible verse when you really need a nap, a hug, or a prescription.
Postpartum depression is not a reflection of your love for your baby. It's a reflection of how much your body has gone through.

Be Gentle With You

Your hormones just went through the biggest shift they'll ever experience. Your body just built, birthed, and is now sustaining a whole human. You don't need to "bounce back." You need time, nourishment, and grace. And space to feel all the things you're feeling.

This part of the journey is still holy. Still feminine. Still deserving of softness. Even when it's messy. Especially when it's messy.

Understanding your reproductive health isn't just about babies—it's about knowing your body and making empowered choices. Whether you're trying to conceive, avoid pregnancy, or just keep your hormones happy, the key is knowledge, balance, and a little bit of control.

And remember: fertility is a team sport. Dads, we see you. Moms, you got this. And for those happily child-free? Keep rocking your life, your way. Your body, your rules.

chapter 7
MANAGING THE UNMANAGABLE

Hormonal imbalances like PCOS (Polycystic Ovary Syndrome) and endometriosis are often brushed off with a dismissive *"just take birth control"* approach. But you deserve more than a prescription and a shrug. These conditions are real. They're complex. They're exhausting. And they can shake your confidence, your energy, and your relationship with your body. With the right knowledge and tools, they're manageable. Let's break it all down so you can take back control of your body.

PCOS

Polycystic Ovary Syndrome (PCOS) isn't just about cysts. It's a hormonal and metabolic condition that affects how your body processes insulin, produces testosterone, and regulates ovulation.
You might be dealing with PCOS if you've noticed:

- Irregular or missing periods
- Unwanted facial or body hair
- Acne that won't go away, no matter what you try
- Sudden or stubborn weight gain
- Thinning hair on your head
- Mood swings, fatigue, or feeling emotionally "off"
- Trouble getting pregnant

Behind the scenes, PCOS usually involves three major issues:

Insulin Resistance
Your body struggles to process insulin properly, which can lead to blood sugar spikes and increased testosterone levels. That combination often causes weight gain, irregular periods, and other hormone chaos.

High Androgens
Elevated "male" hormones can show up as chin hair, hair loss at your temples, jawline breakouts, or feeling disconnected from your femininity.

Inflammation

Many women with PCOS have chronic low-grade inflammation, which only adds fuel to the hormonal fire.

Healing PCOS from the Inside Out

PCOS doesn't have a one-size-fits-all solution—but there are several ways to soothe the storm.

Start with food. Your plate can be your best medicine.

- Stabilize your blood sugar. Every meal should include protein, healthy fat, and fiber. This helps reduce insulin spikes that trigger symptoms.

- Limit dairy and sugar. Both can make inflammation worse and throw hormones further out of balance.

- Focus on real, whole foods. Think: leafy greens, salmon, avocado, nuts, seeds, and root veggies.

Supportive supplements:

- Inositol (Myo & D-Chiro): Great for insulin sensitivity and bringing back regular ovulation.

- Omega-3s: They calm inflammation and help rebalance hormones.

- Spearmint tea: Can naturally lower testosterone and reduce excess hair growth.

- Magnesium & Zinc: Support blood sugar control and ease stress on your system.

Lifestyle:

- Move your body daily, but gently. Strength training, walking, yoga–yes. Overtraining? No. Cortisol spikes can make symptoms worse.

- Prioritize rest. Sleep heals hormones. Period.

- Manage stress like your life depends on it. Because in some ways, it does. Try journaling, breathwork, saying "no," and doing more of what actually makes you feel good.

Endometriosis

Endometriosis is so often misunderstood. It's not "just bad periods." It's when tissue similar to the uterine lining starts growing outside the uterus – sometimes on the ovaries, bladder, bowels, and beyond. It doesn't belong there, and your body knows it.

It can feel like:

- Intense pelvic pain that takes you out of your day
- Pain during or after sex that makes intimacy feel impossible
- Heavy or irregular bleeding
- Bloating so bad you feel six months pregnant
- Fatigue that doesn't go away
- Digestive struggles like constipation, nausea, and diarrhea
- Trouble conceiving, even when you're doing everything "right"

At the root of endo, you'll usually find:

Estrogen dominance
Too much estrogen fuels the growth of that out-of-place tissue.

Systemic inflammation
Your body's immune response is constantly on edge, leading to pain and flare-ups.

Poor detoxification
If your liver isn't clearing hormones properly, things back up fast.

Managing Endo

Pain is real. So is healing. Start with an anti-inflammatory diet. Fill your plate with:

- Leafy greens, berries, and cruciferous vegetables
- Healthy fats like avocado, olive oil, and wild-caught fish
- Anti-inflammatory herbs like turmeric and ginger

Cut back on triggers:
- Dairy
- Gluten
- Processed sugar
- Alcohol

Test what feels good and what flares you up. Keep a journal if it helps.

Supportive supplements:

- Castor oil packs can help soothe inflammation and support lymph flow.

- Acupuncture has been shown to reduce endo pain and help regulate hormones.

- Magnesium + heat = a magic combo for relaxing tense muscles and easing cramps.

Protect your hormones long-term by:

- Reducing exposure to endocrine disruptors (plastics, synthetic fragrances, etc.)

- Supporting your liver with foods like broccoli, kale, and dandelion tea

- Choosing clean beauty and non-toxic cleaning products

- Making time for deep rest, low-stress movement, and connection to yourself

Fibroids

Another condition often overlooked or brushed off as "just heavy periods" is uterine fibroids. These are non-cancerous growths that form in or around the uterus, and they're *extremely* common.

You might be dealing with fibroids if you've experienced:

- Heavy, prolonged periods that leave you drained

- Bloating or a feeling of fullness in your lower belly

- Pelvic pain or pressure

- Frequent peeing or trouble emptying your bladder

- Pain during sex

- Fatigue from low iron (anemia)

Fibroids can range from tiny and harmless to large enough to distort the uterus. And yet, so many women are told to

just wait it out, take iron pills, or "come back when it's worse."

But your suffering doesn't need to reach crisis levels to deserve attention.

Supportive options:

Iron-rich foods & supplements
Especially if you're bleeding heavily and feeling fatigued. Think: spinach, lentils, pumpkin seeds, and liquid iron formulas.

Anti-inflammatory foods
Focus on leafy greens, berries, turmeric, and fatty fish.

Avoid estrogen overload
Limit alcohol, processed soy, and endocrine disruptors like BPA.

Castor oil packs
Gentle, natural support to improve circulation and reduce inflammation.

Vitex (chasteberry)
A hormonal herb that can help regulate cycles and ease symptoms.

Surgery is an option, but not the only one. Uterine-sparing procedures like UFE (Uterine Fibroid Embolization) exist. So do natural approaches. Don't let anyone pressure you into silence or surgery before you feel informed.

Pelvic Floor Dysfunction

This one almost no one prepares us for: the pelvic floor. These are the muscles at the base of your core—supporting your uterus, bladder, bowels, and even your orgasm. But when those muscles become too tight, too weak, or too disconnected, everything from sex to peeing to posture can feel… off.

You might have pelvic floor dysfunction if:

- You leak a little when you sneeze, jump, or laugh
- You feel pressure or heaviness in your pelvis

- You struggle with constipation or incomplete bowel movements

- Sex feels painful, especially at penetration

- You've had birth trauma, pelvic surgery, or chronic stress

This isn't just a "new mom" issue or an "aging" problem. It's a whole-body issue, and it's fixable.

What helps:

Pelvic floor physical therapy
This is the gold standard. A trained therapist can assess muscle strength, tension, and alignment, and give you a personalized recovery plan.

Breathwork & posture
Deep diaphragmatic breathing and learning to relax your pelvic floor is just as important as strengthening it.

Magnesium
Helps calm tight muscles and supports relaxation.

Avoiding over-bracing your core
Sucking in your stomach all day actually weakens your pelvic floor over time.

Tuning into your body
Trauma, shame, and disconnection often live in the pelvis. Healing here is emotional, too.

Adenomyosis

You've probably heard of fibroids and endometriosis, but what about adenomyosis? It's one of the most overlooked reasons why periods can feel like a crime scene and a boxing match rolled into one.

Adenomyosis happens when the same tissue that normally lines your uterus (the endometrium) starts growing into the muscular wall of the uterus. Instead of shedding neatly during your cycle, this tissue gets stuck and causes pain, swelling, and inflammation inside the muscle itself.

You might have adenomyosis if you experience:

- Heavy or prolonged bleeding

- Cramping that feels deep and achy (like it's coming from inside your bones)

- Pelvic pain that lingers between periods

- Pain during sex

- Bloating or a bulging lower belly

- A uterus that feels tender or enlarged

Adenomyosis is tricky because it mimics other conditions, it's often dismissed as "just bad periods" or mistaken for fibroids or endo. But it's its own beast. And like all the rest, it deserves to be taken seriously.

What helps?

Anti-inflammatory Living
Leafy greens, omega-3s, turmeric, ginger, castor oil packs, pelvic steams.

Hormone-balancing Support
Some find relief with hormonal birth control or progestin IUDs to reduce the monthly chaos.

Pain Relief: NSAIDs like ibuprofen can dull the inflammation, but they're not a long-term fix.

Rest and self-compassion
Chronic pain doesn't make you lazy. It makes you resilient.

Some cases of adenomyosis may require surgery if symptoms are severe and persistent. But you have options, and you're not imagining it. If something feels off, keep advocating. Your body always knows.

These conditions may feel unmanageable, but they don't get to own your story.

If you're dealing with PCOS, your path will include balancing blood sugar, calming inflammation, and getting insulin under control. If you're living with endo, it's about easing pain, reducing estrogen overload, and finding sustainable ways to support your body through flare-ups and fatigue. If fibroids are part of your journey, know that you don't have to bleed quietly or suffer in silence. And if your pelvic floor has been screaming for support, trust that healing is possible there, too.

Neither condition defines you. You are not broken. You are not helpless. You are not invisible. You are capable. You are worthy of answers. You are allowed to want more than just symptom control. You're allowed to want to feel whole.

So keep asking questions. Keep trying what feels right for *your* body. And keep honoring the version of you that still shows up, still listens, still hopes—even on the hard days.

You got this.

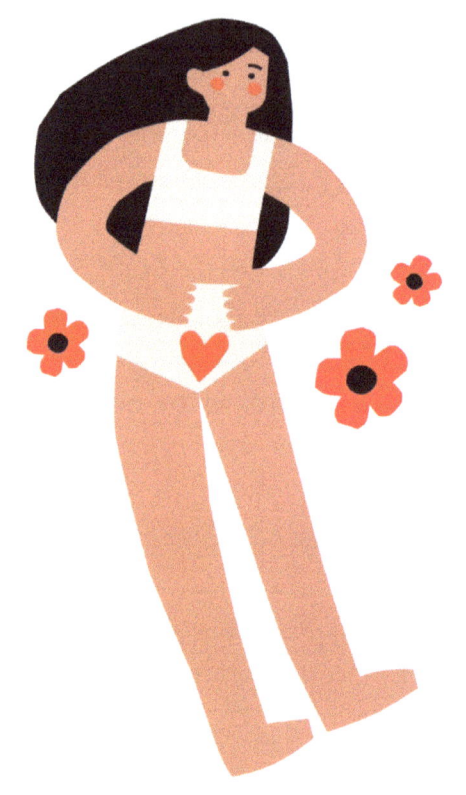

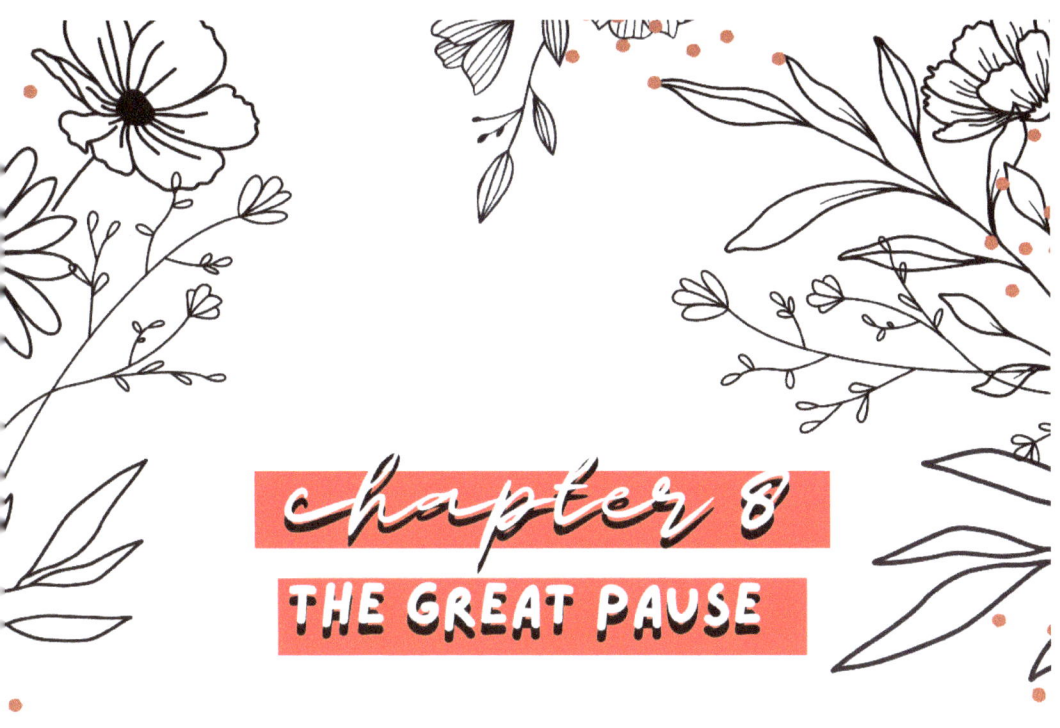

Chapter 8
THE GREAT PAUSE

What if menopause isn't something you survive, but something you emerge from? What if it's the moment you become the version of you that no longer waits for permission? Make no mistake: menopause isn't the end of your youth. It's the beginning of your I-don't-give-a-crap era. Think of it as the ultimate life upgrade. Where your priorities shift, your confidence skyrockets, and you finally stop pretending to care about things that don't serve you.

That said, menopause can also feel like a chaotic rollercoaster ride, and not the fun kind. If you've been feeling like your hormones are playing a cruel joke on you, don't worry, we're about to take the wheel and smooth out this ride.

Perimenopause: The Warm-Up Act

Before menopause officially shows up, there's perimenopause – the messy pre-show that can last anywhere from a few months to a decade. This is when your hormones start playing hopscotch—some months you ovulate, some you don't, and your cycle becomes unpredictable.

Symptoms Can Include:

- Irregular periods (longer, shorter, heavier, lighter)
- Unexplained weight changes
- Brain fog
- Increased anxiety or depression

What Can You Do?

Support Estrogen Naturally
Eat flaxseeds, sesame seeds, and phytoestrogen-rich foods to ease the transition.

Balance Your Blood Sugar
Refined carbs and sugar throw your hormones into chaos.

Lower Cortisol
Chronic stress speeds up hormonal depletion. Try adaptogens, deep breathing, and magnesium.

The Great Pause

Menopause usually crashes the party between ages 45 and 55, marking the official end of your menstrual cycles. It's your body's way of saying, "We're closing up shop – no more monthly visits." The cause? A hormonal shake-up, mainly a drop in estrogen and progesterone, which brings on a delightful mix of symptoms.

Hot Flashes & Night Sweats

You're mid-conversation, and suddenly it feels like your internal thermostat got hijacked. Your face flushes, your chest heats up, and sweat pours from places you didn't know could sweat. Welcome to the fiery chaos of a hot flash. Night sweats? Same thing, just with soaked sheets and 3 a.m. outfit changes.

As estrogen declines, your brain—specifically the hypothalamus (aka your body's thermostat)—becomes more sensitive to slight changes in temperature. This "sensitivity" triggers your body to overreact, thinking you're overheating even when you're not. Cue the flushing, sweating, and sudden chill that follows.

Your blood vessels dilate to release heat (that's the flush), and your sweat glands work overtime to cool you down (that's the drench). Then your body realizes, "Oh… false alarm," and you're left clammy and exhausted.

And yes—cortisol plays a role here too. Stress makes hot flashes worse by destabilizing your nervous system and throwing off your temperature regulation even more.

How to Cool the Flames

Nervous System Regulation
Practice calming techniques like deep breathing, progressive muscle relaxation, or yoga nidra to bring down cortisol and soothe your hypothalamus.

Hydration
Dehydration makes temperature swings worse. Aim for at least half your body weight in ounces of water daily. Add electrolyte-rich drinks if you're sweating often at night.

Cooling Foods & Herbs
Load up on water-dense, cooling foods like cucumber, mint, watermelon, and leafy greens.
Herbs like sage, black cohosh, and red clover have been traditionally used to reduce hot flash frequency and intensity.

Adaptogens
Maca root, ashwagandha, and holy basil support adrenal function and help buffer the hormonal stress response that can trigger hot flashes.

Bedtime Hacks

Wear moisture-wicking sleepwear and use cooling gel pillows or bamboo sheets. Keep a fan or cooling cloth near your bed for those inevitable heat surges.

Track Your Triggers

Alcohol, caffeine, spicy food, sugar, and stress can be major flash fuel. Keep a journal to identify your specific flare-ups.

Insomnia

Let's talk about sleep… or the lack of it. One of the most common (and least respected) symptoms of perimenopause and menopause is disrupted sleep. And not just "I stayed up scrolling" kind of tired. We're talking about wide-awake-at-3am-for-no-reason kind of tired. Exhausted but wired. Brain fog for breakfast.
The culprits? Cortisol, melatonin, and your circadian rhythm – all of which get thrown off as your hormones shift.

- **Cortisol (your stress hormone)** starts peaking at the wrong times, keeping you alert when you're supposed to wind down.

- **Melatonin (your sleep hormone)** starts declining, making it harder to fall and stay asleep.

- **Your circadian rhythm** - the internal clock that once synced like a playlist now feels stuck on shuffle.

What Helps:

- Get sunlight first thing in the morning. It resets your circadian clock and helps melatonin production later.

- Ditch screens 1-2 hours before bed. Blue light delays melatonin release.

- Eat protein-forward dinners with magnesium-rich greens (spinach, chard) to help regulate blood sugar and nervous system calm.

- Try adaptogens like ashwagandha, or magnesium glycinate before bed.

- If cortisol spikes are waking you up early, consider holy basil tea, journaling before bed, and cutting caffeine after noon.

Vaginal Dryness

Nothing about vaginal dryness feels cute. It's uncomfortable, it can make intimacy feel like a chore, and for many women, it's one of the first changes that makes them feel disconnected from their body.
When estrogen drops, so does your body's natural lubrication. The vaginal tissue becomes thinner, less elastic, and more prone to irritation. That doesn't just affect sex – it can impact daily comfort, from wearing leggings to sitting too long.

What Helps:

Vitamin E (topical or suppository)
Acts as a natural moisturizer for the vaginal walls.

Flaxseeds & Omega-3s
These nourish from the inside out and support tissue hydration.

Hyaluronic Acid Suppositories
Yup, the same thing you put on your face can support vaginal tissue.

Phytoestrogens
These plant compounds (like in shatavari, soy, or flax) gently mimic estrogen and can support moisture levels.

Hydration
Your cells can't lubricate if you're dried out from the inside. Water matters more than ever.
If sex is painful—Speak up. Use lube. Not the cheap stuff either—go for water-based, organic or pH-balanced lubes made for sensitive tissues. And if it's deeper than dryness? A pelvic floor therapist or hormone-supportive OB/GYN can help.

Mood Swings

You know the moment when you're crying over a missing sock and five minutes later plotting revenge on your partner for chewing too loud? Yeah — that. Mood swings in menopause aren't "just in your head." They're chemical.

Estrogen plays a huge role in mood regulation. It helps balance serotonin, dopamine, and other neurotransmitters that keep us emotionally steady. When estrogen dips, it's like pulling the rug out from under your brain's emotional support system.

Support Options:

B vitamins (especially B6 & B12)
Support neurotransmitter production and reduce irritability.

Magnesium
Helps regulate mood, ease anxiety, and relax the nervous system.

Adaptogens
Herbs like ashwagandha, rhodiola, or holy basil modulate stress hormones and help you feel emotionally grounded.

Omega-3s
Mood-regulating and inflammation-reducing.

Therapy or support groups
Because you shouldn't have to figure it all out alone.

Your rage, your sadness, your irritability is often a sign that something needs to change. Boundaries. Rest. Support. What looks like a mood swing might be your soul throwing a tantrum because you've been ignoring her for too long.

Bone Density Loss

No one talks about this enough — but bone health is a serious part of menopause. Estrogen doesn't just regulate your cycle and keep your skin plump; it also protects your bones. As estrogen declines, bone breakdown speeds up — putting you at higher risk for osteopenia or osteoporosis.
Support Options:

Strength Training
Lifting weights is your best friend. It stimulates bone growth and builds muscle, which helps prevent falls.

Calcium
Yes, you need it—but preferably from food (like leafy greens, sardines, almonds). If supplementing, make sure it's paired with magnesium and vitamin D.

Vitamin D3 + K2
D3 helps absorb calcium, and K2 ensures it goes to your bones (not your arteries).

Magnesium
Often forgotten, but essential for bone formation and calcium balance.

Collagen
Supports the matrix that bones build upon. Helpful for joints and skin, too.

Bone density scans are worth it—especially if menopause hits early or you have a family history of fractures or osteoporosis. And here's the empowering piece: You are not fragile. You are rebuilding. You are reinforcing the very framework that holds your powerful body together. One weight, one walk, one plate of greens at a time—you're reclaiming strength from the inside out.

Brain Fog

You walk into a room and immediately forget why you're there. You open your mouth and the word just… disappears. You reread the same sentence three times and still don't know what you just read. That's not early dementia – that's hormone-driven brain fog.

During perimenopause and menopause, your estrogen levels don't just drop—they fluctuate like a chaotic stock market. Estrogen affects memory, concentration, and verbal processing. So when it's out of whack, your brain feels like it's running on dial-up in a 5G world.

Estrogen Decline
Estrogen supports neurotransmitters like serotonin, dopamine, and acetylcholine, which are crucial for memory and mood. Less estrogen = slower mental processing.

Poor Sleep
If you're tossing and turning all night, your brain doesn't get time to organize and reset. Cue the morning fog.

Cortisol Overload
Stress hijacks focus. Elevated cortisol literally pulls blood flow away from the brain and toward "fight or flight" mode.

Blood Sugar Swings
Your brain thrives on stable glucose. Sudden drops from skipping meals or carb crashes can make your thoughts feel like molasses.

Support Options:

Protein & Healthy Fats
Fuel your brain with foods that don't spike blood sugar. Eggs, salmon, nuts, avocado, chia seeds.

B Vitamins & Omega-3s
B-complex vitamins (especially B6, B9, and B12) support cognitive function. Omega-3s reduce inflammation and keep your brain sharp.

Lion's Mane & Ginkgo Biloba
These herbs support neuroplasticity and circulation to the brain.

Cognitive Routines
Brain fog hates structure. Try simple lists, check-ins, and using phone reminders like breadcrumbs.

Sleep & Stress Reduction
You can't out-supplement a fried nervous system. Meditate. Breathe. Nap if you need to.

You're not losing your mind—your hormones are just playing musical chairs. You're still brilliant, still capable, and still YOU. Your brain might be recalibrating, but trust—she's still in there.

Beyond the Symptoms

Menopause changes how we look and how we feel. Our bodies shift, our desires evolve, and suddenly we're navigating uncharted waters — sometimes with partners who don't know how to meet us there.

But here's what I want you to know: Your pleasure doesn't expire. Your sex appeal doesn't have an age limit. And your need for emotional connection deepens, not disappears.

The Role of Emotional Intimacy & Body Confidence

Menopause does not mean your sex life is over. In fact, it can mean quite the opposite. When you're no longer on the hormonal rollercoaster of cycling every month, you have the chance to rebuild your relationship with pleasure on your terms. Slower. Softer. Wilder. Whatever your body craves now.

Many women report better sex post-menopause because it's no longer about performance or people-pleasing. It's about presence, sensation, and connection. That said, changes in hormones do affect libido, moisture, and arousal patterns, so here's how to keep that fire burning.

Foreplay isn't optional – it's the main course.
With less estrogen, natural lubrication and arousal may take more time. That's not a flaw. That's your body inviting you to slow down.

Lube is self-care.
Choose organic, water- or aloe-based lubes without glycerin (which can cause irritation).

Try vaginal moisturizers.
Not just lube – we're talking daily hydration for vaginal tissues. Products with hyaluronic acid or vitamin E can work wonders.

Reframe sex.
It doesn't have to look how it used to. Think sensual touch, massage, mutual pleasure, toys, exploration. There are no rules, only options.

Confidence isn't about looking the same, it's about feeling at home in your skin. And emotional intimacy? It starts with *you*. When you show up with self-awareness, clarity, and softness, you create a space where real connection thrives.

When Menopause Comes Early

Menopause before 45 is considered early, and before 40 it's called Premature Ovarian Insufficiency (POI). If your cycle is MIA too soon, there's probably an underlying cause.
Why It Might Happen:

Chronic Stress & Burnout
Running on adrenaline and caffeine can exhaust your hormones.

Autoimmune Disorders
Sometimes your immune system mistakenly attacks your ovaries.

Genetics

If your mom or grandma experienced early menopause, you might be predisposed too.

Thyroid & Metabolic Issues

A sluggish thyroid can mess with your menstrual cycle.

Toxins & Endocrine Disruptors

Plastics, pesticides, and synthetic hormones disrupt ovarian function.

How to Support or Slow Early Menopause

Support Your Adrenals

Ashwagandha, magnesium, and rest can help keep cortisol in check.

Eat Estrogen-Loving Foods

Flaxseeds, sesame seeds, fermented soy, and leafy greens are your friends.

Balance Your Blood Sugar

Stabilize glucose with protein, fiber, and healthy fats.

Correct Deficiencies

Low vitamin D, iron, B vitamins, or omega-3s can impact your hormones.

Reduce Toxins
Switch to clean beauty products, non-toxic cleaning, and filtered water.

Get Hormone Testing
Especially if you're under 45 and experiencing symptoms. Ask about FSH, AMH, and estrogen levels.

When You Start Questioning Yourself

Menopause doesn't just change your body—it can shake your sense of identity. The world doesn't talk enough about what it means to shift from "fertile and youthful" to "wise and powerful." That shift can feel lonely, invisible, or disorienting. You may wonder: *Who am I now?*

This is your reminder: You're still YOU – just deeper, wiser, freer. Maybe for the first time in your life, your worth doesn't revolve around how much you give, how "desirable" you appear, or how well you hold everything together.

Let your identity stretch. Let your body evolve. Let yourself bloom in ways you never knew were possible.

Advocating for Yourself

If you've ever been told "it's just menopause," or brushed off when describing your pain, you're not imagining it. Women are more likely to be dismissed, misdiagnosed, or told to just "lose weight and relax."

Here's how to protect your power:

- Come to appointments with a written list of symptoms, questions, and goals

- Track your cycle, sleep, energy, and mood shifts to bring data, not just "feelings"

- Ask for specific labs: FSH, LH, estradiol, progesterone, thyroid panel, vitamin D, and iron

- If you're not being heard? Say: "I don't feel like my concerns are being taken seriously. I'd like to explore further options or speak to someone more experienced in menopause care."

- Don't settle for a provider who dismisses you. Your health is not a debate.

Menopause isn't a diagnosis, it's a transition. And you deserve to be met with support, not silence.

Aging in a woman's body comes with whispers, warnings, and shame—as if menopause is the beginning of the end. But it's not the end of your relevance, your sexiness, your ambition, or your vitality. It's just the end of your reproductive years—not the end of your *power*.

We've been taught to shrink as we age. To disappear. But the truth is, many women don't even come fully *into* themselves until after 40.

Menopause isn't a curse. It's a clearing. Let's retire the shame and rewrite the story.

chapter 9
TRUST YOUR GUT

Your hormones and your gut? BFFs. Ride-or-die partners. They're so interconnected that when one goes rogue, the other follows. So if your digestion is all over the place—bloating, breakouts, and random mood swings—you can bet your hormones are throwing a tantrum, too.

Think of your gut as the control center for your body. It's where nutrients are absorbed, hormones are metabolized, and detoxification happens. When your gut is happy, your hormones are balanced. When it's pissed off? You get acne, mood swings, bloating, brain fog, period drama, and that general "ugh, I feel off" vibe.

The good news? You have a lot more control over this than you think. Let's get into the gut-hormone gossip so you can start healing from the inside out.

How Your Gut Affects Your Hormones

Your gut and hormones talk to each other all day long. The problem is, if your gut is inflamed, sluggish, or overloaded with junk, that convo is full of mixed signals. Your gut is supposed to break down food, absorb nutrients, and clear out excess hormones. But if it's overburdened, those hormones don't leave the way they should—and instead, they recycle back into your system like an ex that just won't quit.

And then, of course, all hell breaks loose.

Signs Your Gut is Wrecking Your Hormones:

- Bloating that makes you look three months pregnant (even when all you had was a salad)

- Breakouts that won't quit, no matter how many skincare products you try

- PMS from the depths of hell - cramps, mood swings, heavy bleeding

- Unpredictable cycles (your period should not be showing up like an uninvited guest)

- Fatigue, brain fog, and feeling generally meh

- Digestive drama – constipation, diarrhea, or both (lucky you!)

Bad Gut Equals Bad Periods

Your period should not be a monthly horror movie. If you're bloating, cramping, breaking out, or having mood swings that scare small children, it's time to check in with your gut.

Why? Because your gut is in charge of eliminating old estrogen. If it's backed up, inflamed, or full of bad bacteria, that estrogen sticks around too long, causing heavier periods, crazy PMS, and mood swings that make no sense.

But don't worry—this isn't a life sentence. Healing your gut equals happier, healthier, more balanced hormones.

Foods That Feed Your Gut

Time to ditch the gut-wrecking foods (lookin' at you, processed junk and excess sugar) and bring in the good stuff. Your gut needs fiber, probiotics, and anti-inflammatory foods to keep digestion smooth, balance hormones, and make you feel amazing.

The Gut-Healing Grocery List

Fiber is Queen
Found in leafy greens, flaxseeds, chia seeds, apples, and oats, fiber keeps things moving (which we'll talk about more in a sec). Bonus? It also feeds your good gut bacteria, making your microbiome happy and thriving.

Probiotics
Your Gut's Best Friend – Good bacteria = happy gut. Get yours from yogurt (if you tolerate dairy), sauerkraut, kimchi, kefir, miso, and kombucha. These fermented foods help your gut break down food, absorb nutrients, and get rid of excess estrogen.

Liver-Loving Foods
Your liver is the detox powerhouse that helps clear out used hormones. Lemon water, cruciferous veggies (broccoli, Brussels sprouts, cabbage), turmeric, and dandelion root tea all give it a boost.

Healthy Fats
For Hormone Production – Avocados, olive oil, salmon, nuts, and seeds support hormone production and reduce inflammation. (Yes, you can eat fat without fear—it's not 1995 anymore).

Cut the Gut Killers
Processed sugar, artificial sweeteners, and excessive dairy inflame your gut, disrupt your hormones, and make PMS worse. If you're still drinking diet soda, consider this your sign to break up.

Poop Talk:

Yep, we're going there. Because if you're constipated, your hormones are, too.

Estrogen, once it's done doing its thing, is supposed to be escorted out of your body via your liver and intestines. But if you're not pooping daily, that estrogen just sits in your gut and gets reabsorbed—leading to PMS, mood swings, acne, and heavier periods.

So, yeah, pooping is a non-negotiable part of hormone balance.

Signs You Need to Get Things Moving:

- You don't go at least once a day

- Your poop is hard, dry, or feels like giving birth to a small boulder

- You feel bloated, sluggish, or constantly full

- You know you need to go, but nothing happens (ugh)

How to Fix It:

Eat more fiber
Flaxseeds, veggies, fruits, whole grains – fiber keeps things moving.

Drink more water
Yes, it matters. Hydration = smoother exits

Magnesium citrate
This mineral is a game changer for getting things moving

Move your body
Exercise stimulates digestion, so take that walk

Support Detox Pathways
Help your liver clear out old hormones with cruciferous veggies, dandelion tea, and fiber

Castor oil packs
Sounds weird, but rubbing castor oil on your abdomen can help stimulate digestion & detox your liver

Repopulate with Good Bacteria
Load up on fermented foods and a quality probiotic to support digestion and hormone balance

Heal Your Gut Lining
Cut inflammatory foods (processed sugar, gluten, excessive dairy) and focus on whole, gut-friendly foods.

Your gut is the foundation of your hormonal health. If you're bloated, constipated, moody, breaking out, or experiencing period chaos, start with your digestion.

By healing your gut, balancing your microbiome, and keeping things moving, you're setting yourself up for hormonal harmony, glowing skin, and smooth cycles.

It's not about perfection, it's about supporting your body in ways that actually work. So, grab that kombucha, eat your fiber, and make daily poops a priority—your hormones will thank you.

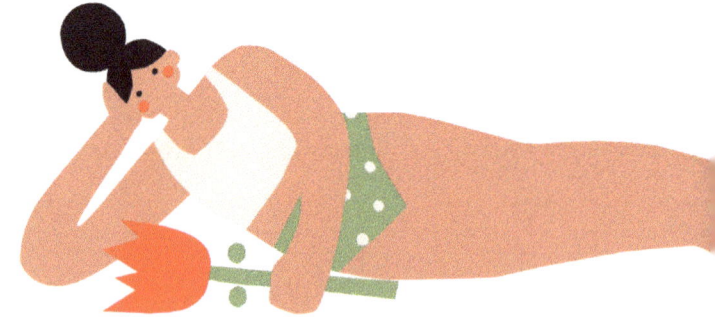

Chapter 10
THE BEAUTY BLUEPRINT

Ever wondered why your skin is staging a rebellion, your hair is thinning faster than your patience, or your body just feels off? These aren't just random annoyances. They're messages from your body. Your hormones, gut health, nutrition, and stress levels all play a role in how you look and feel.

Let's decode those messages, fix the root causes, and finally get that glowing skin, thick hair, and vibrant energy you deserve.

Acne & Breakouts

Just so we're clear: hormonal acne is NOT just a teenage thing. If your skin flares up around your jawline, chin, or back, it's usually hormonal—not just bad luck.

The Acne Culprits:

DHT & Androgens
High-testosterone troublemakers, causing deep, cystic acne, especially in PCOS or hormonal imbalances.

Inflammation Overload
Dairy, sugar, and gut imbalances are major acne triggers.

Poor Detox Pathways
If your liver isn't detoxing properly, extra hormones and toxins get dumped into your skin—causing breakouts.

Estrogen Dominance or Progesterone Deficiency - When these hormones aren't balanced, your skin can become oily, acne-prone, or extra sensitive.

How to Fix It:

Balance Androgens Naturally

- Spearmint tea (2 cups a day) helps lower testosterone-driven acne.

- Zinc & Omega-3s reduce inflammation and help skin heal faster.

- Cut back on dairy & sugar—they spike insulin and make acne worse.

Support Your Skin's Detox Pathways

- Liver-loving foods: Lemon water, cruciferous veggies, and dandelion tea flush out excess hormones.

- Hydration is key. Drink plenty of water to clear skin-damaging toxins.

- Poop daily. If you're constipated, old hormones get reabsorbed—and show up on your face.

Topical Support That Works:

- Azelaic acid & niacinamide calm inflammation and fade dark spots.

- Salicylic acid unclogs pores and reduces oil production.

- Gentle cleansing only. Over-cleansing strips your skin and makes oil production worse.

Dry Skin SOS

Your skin isn't just thirsty for lotion—it wants nourishment, hydration, and a strong barrier.

Hydration Starts Inside

- Water alone isn't enough. Add electrolytes (like sea salt + lemon or coconut water) to help your cells absorb moisture.

- Eat healthy fats: avocado, olive oil, nuts, seeds, and fatty fish lock in skin moisture.

Nourish Your Skin Barrier

- Topical ceramides, colloidal oats, and squalane help restore your skin's protective barrier.

- Use gentle cleansers, not harsh foaming ones.

- Seal in moisture with an occlusive like shea butter or balm after your body cream.

- Dry Skin Heroes
    - Omega-3s (from fish oil or flax)
    - Vitamin E (skin repair)
    - Aloe vera (hydrating + soothing)

Hair Loss & Thinning

Hair loss is a gut punch. Whether you're losing it in handfuls, noticing thinning around your part, or dealing with a receding hairline, it's not just a hair problem, it's a health problem. Your hair is an extension of your body's nutrient stores. So if you're shedding like crazy, your body is waving a red flag.

Common Causes of Hair Loss:

Low Iron & Ferritin
If your iron levels are low, your hair stops growing and starts falling out. (*Heavy periods? You're likely iron deficient.*)

Thyroid Imbalances
Slow thyroid = slow hair growth + excessive shedding. If you're cold all the time, exhausted, or gaining weight out of nowhere, get your thyroid checked.

Protein Deficiency
Hair is made of protein. If you're not eating enough, your hair gets weak, brittle, and thin.

Inflammation & Stress
Chronic stress raises cortisol, which shrinks your hair follicles (*rude*). Inflammation disrupts hair growth cycles, causing premature shedding.

Hormonal Imbalances
High androgens (hello, PCOS!) or low progesterone can lead to thinning hair & hairline recession.

How to Get Your Hair Back:

Iron + Biotin + Collagen
Your hair's best friends.

- Iron (with vitamin C!) supports oxygen flow to your scalp & hair follicles.

- **Biotin** strengthens hair (*but only works if you're already getting enough nutrients*).

- Collagen (or bone broth) boosts scalp health and keratin production.

Scalp Care
Rosemary oil, castor oil scalp massages, and gentle haircare can stimulate blood flow and encourage regrowth.'

- Peppermint oil (diluted) can stimulate circulation even more effectively than minoxidil in some studies.

- Microneedling or derma-rolling the scalp (safely!) creates micro-injuries that boost collagen and improve absorption of oils or serums.
- Inversion method (flipping your head upside down for 2-4 minutes during scalp massage) may increase blood flow to follicles.

Gut & Nutrient Absorption

You can eat all the right things, but if your gut isn't absorbing nutrients properly, your hair will still suffer.

- Consider a probiotic and digestive enzyme routine.

- Check for zinc and vitamin D deficiencies—both are crucial for hair growth.

- Eliminate inflammatory foods if you suspect leaky gut or autoimmune flares (especially for conditions like alopecia areata).

Gentle, Protective Hair Habits

- Sleep on silk pillowcases.

- Use satin scrunchies instead of tight elastics.

- Protective styles matter—especially for textured hair. Avoid too-tight braids, wigs with tension, or daily heat styling.

- Wash less frequently (1-2x/week), and use a clarifying rinse (like apple cider vinegar) monthly.

Hormone Balancing

If hair loss is tied to PCOS, postpartum shifts, thyroid imbalances, or perimenopause, no amount of biotin will fix it until hormones are rebalanced.

- Adaptogens like *ashwagandha* and *maca* may support hormonal equilibrium.

- Get your thyroid and ferritin levels tested—especially if you've had a baby or have irregular cycles.

- Consider saw palmetto (blocks DHT) for androgen-related hair loss.

Strengthen Your Nails

Weak, peeling, or brittle nails are often more than cosmetic—they're little messengers showing you what's happening inside.

Nutrients That Feed Your Nails

Biotin
Supports keratin infrastructure. (You'll find it in eggs, nuts, and biotin-rich supplements.)

Silica
Found in horsetail extract and cucumber, helps with nail strength and flexibility.

Iron + B12
Thin, spoon-shaped, or pale nails? Could be low iron or B12.

Zinc
Prevents white spots and supports tissue repair.

Garlic for Growth
It sounds wild, but it works. Garlic is antimicrobial and rich in selenium. Rub raw garlic juice or garlic oil into your cuticles 2-3x/week or look for nail strengtheners infused with garlic extract. (Bonus: it helps kill nail fungus, too.)

Protect & Hydrate
Keep nails short and rounded if they split easily.
Moisturize cuticles with jojoba oil, shea butter, or vitamin E.
Avoid acetone-based polish removers, which strip oils and dry the nail plate.

Naturally Beat Body Odor

Your sweat isn't the problem, it's the bacteria that feed on it. And yes, you can smell like a queen without a single drop of aluminum-laced deodorant.

Natural Body Odor Hacks

Lime or lemon slices
Wipe underarms with fresh citrus to kill odor-causing bacteria.

Coconut oil
Naturally antimicrobial. Use as a base layer before natural deodorant.

Baking Soda + Arrowroot
Mix with a little coconut oil for a simple DIY paste.

Chlorophyll Supplements
Help from the inside out by reducing odor-causing compounds.

Probiotic-Rich Foods
Like sauerkraut, kefir, or kombucha—support a healthier skin microbiome.

How to Smell Like a Goddess

The secret isn't just the perfume, it's the ritual. Here's your signature scent layering routine for smelling divine all day long.

Wash in Layers

- Start with antibacterial soap to remove odor-causing bacteria (especially in sweat zones).

- If it's hair wash day, wash your hair first—otherwise, that shampoo runoff is just clinging to clean skin.

- Use an African net sponge—it exfoliates better than a loofah and doesn't harbor bacteria.

- After rinsing, use your scented body wash—the one that makes you feel like a snack.

- Gently cleanse your yoni with water or a pH-friendly wash—skip harsh soaps.

- Use a separate cloth for your booty. (Because... hygiene.)

- Shave or exfoliate where needed. Exfoliating before shaving helps with ingrowns and smoothness.

Lock It In Post-Shower

- While damp, apply a matching-scented lotion or body cream. This helps the scent linger.

- Layer with a body spray or perfume in the same fragrance family. Hit pulse points: neck, wrists, behind knees.

- Toss a mini perfume in your bag for touch-ups.

Your skin, hair, and body are constantly giving you clues about what's happening internally. If you're dealing with breakouts, hair loss, or dryness, it's time to look beyond quick fixes and treat the root cause.

Your health and beauty go hand in hand. Nourish your body, listen to what it needs, and let your natural glow shine through.

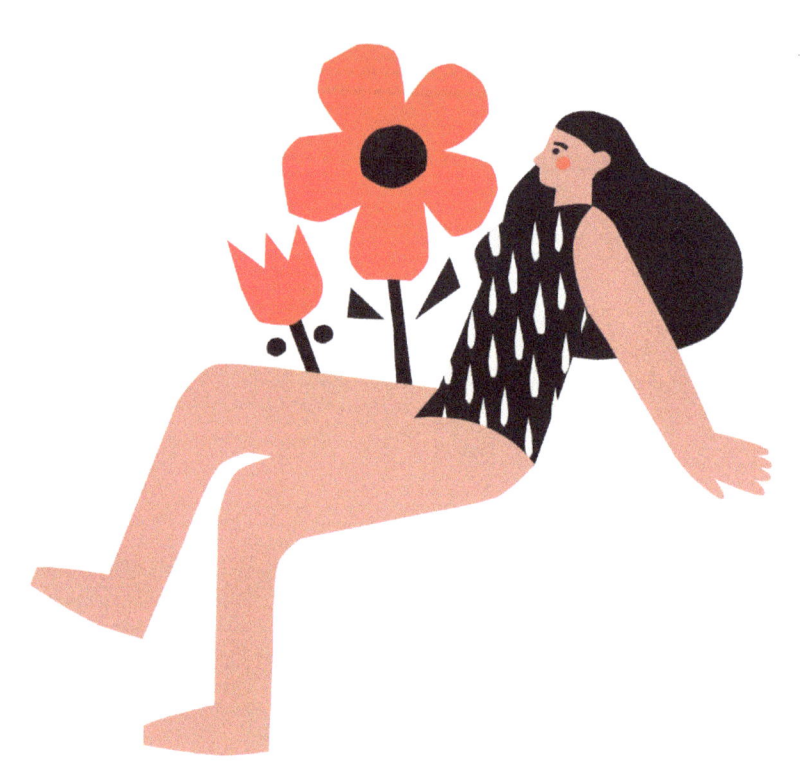

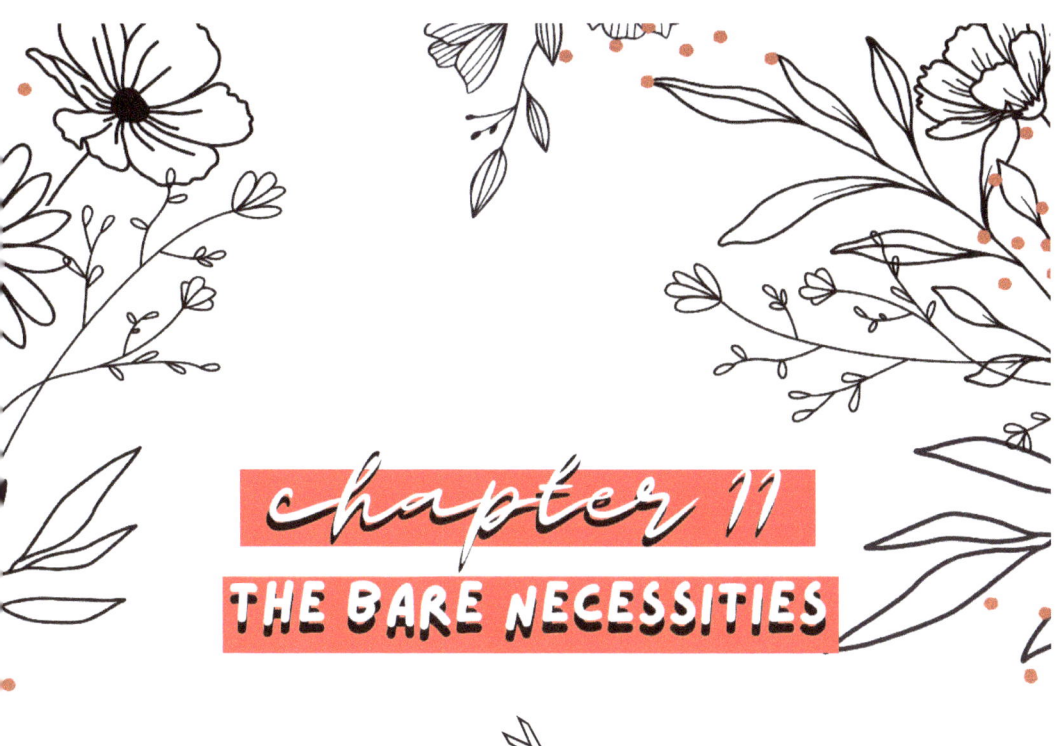

Chapter 11
THE BARE NECESSITIES

Ah, shaving. The fine art of shearing your lady garden. The timeless ritual of dragging a tiny, angry blade across your skin in the hopes of achieving goddess-level smoothness. The ultimate test of patience, precision, and pain tolerance. But fear not, because today, we're reclaiming the razor and turning it into a tool of empowerment—without the trauma of razor burn, ingrown hairs, or that one awkward patch you always seem to miss.

And listen, hair removal is optional. If you love the smooth life, go for it. If you want to let your leg hair flow in the wind, that's also iconic. The only rule? Do whatever makes *you* feel good. But if you're going to shave, at least do it with the right tools, the right technique, and the right mindset (which is: expect chaos, but hope for smoothness).

What's your She-Weapon of Choice?

Not all razors are created equal, my dear smooth-seekers. Drugstore pink razors? Absolute trash. They dull faster than a toddler's safety scissors and cost twice as much as the men's version. Go figure. Instead, we're talking about high-quality, skin-loving tools that glide like a dream and don't play you like a fool.

Safety Razors
Old-school, sleek, and intimidating as hell, but once you get the hang of them, they deliver a close, irritation-free shave that's practically meditative.

Electric Shavers
The lazy girl's dream. Less risk, less drama, but you won't get that ultra-silky dolphin skin effect. Perfect for touch-ups and quick deforestation.

Multi-Blade Razors
They'll give you that butter-smooth finish but can also increase irritation and those cursed ingrowns if not handled with care.

Set Yourself Up for Shaving Glory

Your skin is not a dry erase board, and razors are not meant to be dragged across it willy-nilly. Let's prep properly.

Get Wet
A warm shower or bath softens the hair and opens up the pores, making the entire process way less painful. Dry shaving? Only if you like suffering.

Exfoliate
A good scrub before you shave removes dead skin cells and helps prevent those sneaky little ingrowns from ruining your life.

Slather Up
Shaving cream, oil, conditioner—whatever makes your razor glide smoothly. Dry skin and friction are a recipe for disaster.

The Stroke of Genius

Now, onto the actual act of shaving, which is basically a strategic game of 'How Not to Slice Yourself.'

Go with the grain first.
It's tempting to go against the grain immediately for that extra-close shave, but that's how you summon the demons of irritation and bumps. Start with the hair growth, then go against it if necessary.

Short, gentle strokes.
No need to bulldoze your skin—your razor is sharp, and your skin is sensitive. Show some love.

Rinse frequently
A clogged razor is a useless razor. Keep it fresh, keep it clean.

Avoiding the Razor Rage

You're smoother than a baby's bottom and feeling yourself. But hold up—don't skip the aftercare.

Cool Rinse
Splash your skin with cold water to close those pores and calm any inflammation.

Moisturize
Preferably with something soothing, like aloe vera, shea butter, coconut oil (great for preventing ingrowns), or your favorite non-comedogenic oil like jojoba or grapeseed. These lock in moisture, calm inflammation, and keep your skin silky—not bumpy.

Avoid Tight Clothes
Give your skin some breathing room. The last thing you need is friction undoing all your hard work.

The Great Ingrown Hair Battle

Ingrown hairs are those rude little reminders that your follicles have minds of their own. Here's how to keep them from staging a mutiny:

- Exfoliate regularly to prevent hairs from getting trapped under the skin.

- Use a gentle acid (like salicylic or glycolic) to keep pores clear.

- Don't pick at them! Let them rise to the surface like the dramatic attention-seekers they are.

Waxing Hair Removal Method

Waxing is for the brave. The bold. The ones willing to trade 10 seconds of pure agony for weeks of smoothness. It's the ultimate "rip the bandage off" approach to hair removal.

The Emotional Stages of Waxing

- **Confidence** – *"I got this. I'm tired of shaving every two days. I'm gonna wax, and it's gonna be amazing."*

- **Doubt** - *"Wait… how much is this gonna hurt?"*

- **Regret** - *First strip gets pulled. You ascend to another dimension.*

- **Acceptance** - *You're already here, so you might as well finish the job.*

- **Euphoria** - *Once the pain fades, you realize you're smoother than a dolphin, and suddenly, it all feels worth it.*

Why Waxing is Both the Best and Worst Thing Ever

The Good:

- Lasts *weeks* instead of days (yes, weeks—shaving could never).

- Hair grows back finer and softer over time.

- No razor burn, no accidental gashes, no 5 o'clock shadow.

- Your skin feels like a *baby seal* when it's done right.

The Bad:

- It hurts. (Some areas worse than others, but… yeah, it's *not* a spa day.)
- It's messy. If you've ever tried an at-home waxing kit, you know the wax gets everywhere and somehow stays sticky *forever.*

- If you're not careful, *hello, ingrown hairs*.

Verdict? If you can handle the pain and want low maintenance, waxing wins. If you like convenience and have a low pain tolerance, shaving is your safe space.

Tips for Waxing Like a Pro

Before Waxing:

- Exfoliate the night before—dead skin = ingrown hairs waiting to happen.

- Take a painkiller 30 minutes before (*because, trust me, you'll thank yourself*).

- If you're DIYing it, make sure your hair is the right length—about a grain of rice long (too short, and the wax won't grab it; too long, and you'll be *screaming*).

During Waxing:

- Hold your skin taut (loose skin = *more pain*).

- Rip the strip off like you mean it—slowly peeling it is *actual torture*.
- Breathe through it. (*Deep breaths. Cry if you need to. You'll survive.*)

After Waxing:

- Moisturize with aloe or fragrance-free lotion. Your skin is *traumatized*—be nice to it.

- Avoid tight clothing for a day (your freshly waxed skin needs *space*).

- Exfoliate gently after a few days to prevent ingrown hairs.

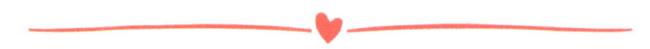

So… What's the right hair removal method for you? Honestly? It depends on your vibe. If you love instant results and don't mind frequent upkeep: Shaving is your girl. If you'd rather suffer once for weeks of smoothness: Waxing is the way. If you never want to deal with this again: keep it natural, babe.

With the right tools, prep, and aftercare, you can achieve silky, irritation-free skin without losing your sanity (or your dignity). Now, go forth and glide, you magnificent, smooth-skinned queen! May your shave be close, your skin be soft, and your knees remain intact.

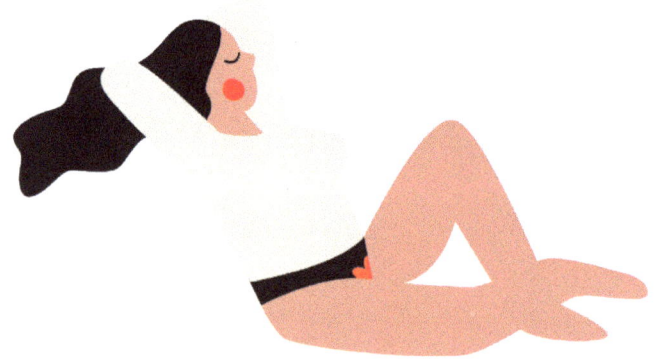

chapter 12
STRESS? I DON'T KNOW HER

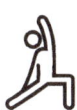

Stress: the modern plague. It's everywhere — hiding in emails, to-do lists, screaming kids, traffic jams, unrealistic expectations, and the people who text "can I call you real quick?" like it's not a trap.

We live in a world where being busy is a badge of honor and burnout is basically an expectation. But chronic stress is an absolute hormone wrecker. It's the reason your periods are unpredictable, your belly is bloated, your sleep is trash, and your mood swings make you question your own sanity.

So, how do we stop stress from turning us into frazzled, exhausted, anxiety-ridden gremlins? Let's break it down.

Why Cortisol is Running the Show

Cortisol isn't the bad guy. She's your "get-up-and-survive" hormone. The one that helps you focus, get out of bed, and respond to real danger. But when life becomes a non-stop emergency—from toxic relationships to overpacked schedules to your own inner critic—cortisol doesn't shut off.

That's when she turns from helpful to hostile:

Steals From Progesterone
Messing up your cycles, amplifying PMS, and leaving you tense, anxious, or weepy.

Spikes Blood Sugar
Triggering cravings, mood swings, and stubborn belly weight.

Ruins Sleep
Especially when it peaks at 2 or 3 a.m. and leaves you tired but wired.

Wrecks Digestion
Because your body doesn't care about digesting lunch when it thinks you're in danger. Cue bloating, gas, or constipation. If your brain feels scattered, your gut is off, your patience is gone, and your period is a whole mess— cortisol may be behind it.

Signs Cortisol is Wrecking Your Life

- You're exhausted but can't relax

- You crave sugar, caffeine, or chips constantly

- You're gaining weight (especially around your waist)

- You have random bursts of irritation or anxiety

- You keep waking up in the middle of the night

- Your brain is foggy

- Your period is irregular, missing, or extra intense

How to Lower Cortisol

You don't have to escape to a remote island to lower your stress. Small, consistent habits can bring your hormones back into balance and help you feel like a functioning human again.

Adaptogens

Adaptogens are herbs that help your body *adapt* to stress. They don't numb you – they nourish you.

Ashwagandha
Calms anxiety, helps with sleep, supports thyroid and adrenals.

Rhodiola
Great if you feel drained and unmotivated. Reboots energy without the crash.

Holy Basil (Tulsi)
Balances blood sugar and soothes frazzled nerves.

Reishi Mushroom
A nervous system hug in mushroom form. Great for winding down.

Give them a few weeks to work. You're not numbing the problem – you're building resilience.

Breathwork

The reset button in your lungs. One of the quickest ways to send your body the message "you're safe" is to slow your breath. Seriously. That's it.

Box Breathing:

- Inhale for 4
- Hold for 4
- Exhale for 4
- Hold for 4

Repeat until your shoulders drop and your brain slows down. Even 2 minutes can shift your whole chemistry.

Move Your Body

Not all workouts are stress-reducing – some actually spike cortisol higher (looking at you, excessive HIIT).

Best workouts for balancing cortisol:

Walking
20-30 minutes a day is magic for stress.

Yoga or Pilates
Lowers cortisol + improves flexibility = double win.

Strength Training
Muscle = better metabolism = happier hormones. Avoid excessive cardio if you're already feeling burnt out—it can make stress and hormone imbalances worse.

Magnesium

Magnesium is basically nature's Xanax. If you're feeling anxious, wired, or waking up at 3 AM for no reason, you need more magnesium.

Best types:

- **Magnesium Glycinate** – Best for stress, anxiety, and better sleep.

- **Magnesium Citrate** – Helps digestion and constipation.

- **Magnesium L-Threonate** – Brain booster! Helps memory + mental clarity.

Prioritize Sleep

If you're not sleeping well, you're not healing. Period. Poor sleep = higher cortisol, more cravings, bad moods, and hormone imbalances.

Better Sleep Hacks:

- Blue-light blocking glasses after sunset = better melatonin production.

- Cut caffeine after 2 PM (yes, even if you think you're "fine").

- Ashwagandha + Magnesium = The ultimate sleep combo.

- Cool bedroom, blackout curtains, and no scrolling before bed.

Stress isn't just a feeling. It's a hormone disrupter, period destroyer, gut wrecker, and metabolism killer. If you've been running on fumes, pushing through exhaustion, and running on caffeine and adrenaline, it's time to reset. Lowering cortisol = better energy, stable moods, deep sleep, clearer skin, and balanced hormones.

Your body is not a machine—you are not supposed to be in a constant state of stress. Start supporting your nervous system, lower that cortisol, and take your power back.

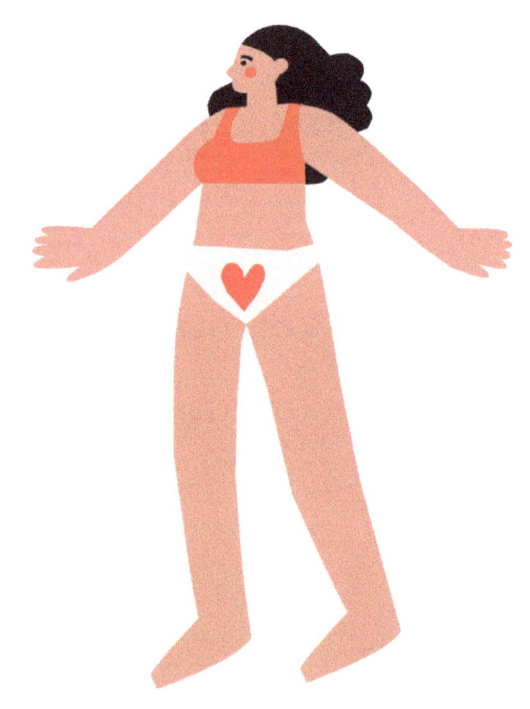

chapter 13
FLUSHING OUT THE FUNK

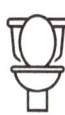

Detox. The word alone probably makes you think of sad green juices, expensive "cleanses," and influencers swearing by celery water at sunrise. But real detox? It's not about starving yourself or drinking something that tastes like lawn clippings. Detox isn't punishment. It's restoration. It's love. It's giving your body the tools it needs to release what no longer serves.

Your body is already detoxing every single day. Your liver, kidneys, gut, skin, and lymphatic system are constantly processing what you eat, breathe, touch, and feel. But we live in a toxic world. And those systems? They're overwhelmed. That's where you come in. Not with extremes, but with intention.

If your skin is breaking out, your digestion is sluggish, or your periods are acting brand new…

If you feel bloated, foggy, inflamed, exhausted, or just *off*…

Then your body might be begging for a gentle, hormone-friendly reset. And no, we're not talking about those awful "7-day cleanses" that leave you starving and miserable. This is about nourishing your body, loving your liver, and actually supporting detox the way nature intended.

Love Your Liver

Detox starts and ends with your liver. This powerhouse organ is your body's ultimate filter—working hard to process hormones, clear out toxins, and flush out waste. But when it's overloaded with processed foods, alcohol, stress, and environmental toxins? Your hormones get backed up, leading to breakouts, bloating, heavy periods, and feeling like a hormonal hot mess.

Liver Love 101

Eat Your Cruciferous Veggies
Broccoli, cauliflower, Brussels sprouts, kale, and cabbage help your liver break down excess estrogen (which is key for hormone balance).

Start Your Day with Lemon Water
Supports digestion and flushes toxins through the liver. Bonus: It wakes up your metabolism and helps with bloating.

Dandelion Root Tea & Milk Thistle
These herbs are liver MVPs. Dandelion root supports bile production and digestion, while milk thistle protects and regenerates liver cells.

Healthy Fats
Avocados, olive oil, flaxseeds, and nuts help your liver process fat-soluble toxins. Plus, they're great for hormone health!

Hydrate
Water flushes out toxins through urine, sweat, and digestion. Aim for at least half your body weight in ounces daily (and no, coffee doesn't count).

Toxins to Avoid

Toxins are everywhere (annoying, right?). They sneak into our food, beauty products, and even the air we breathe. But the worst part? Many of them are hormone disruptors, meaning they mess with estrogen, progesterone, and testosterone, throwing everything off balance.

Plastics & BPA

Found in water bottles, food containers, and receipts (yes, even touching receipts can transfer BPA into your system). Switch to glass, stainless steel, or BPA-free alternatives.

Conventional Tampons & Pads

Many brands contain pesticides, chlorine, and synthetic fragrances that can irritate your vaginal microbiome. Switch to organic cotton, menstrual cups, or period underwear.

Fragrance & Perfume

If it says "fragrance" on the label, it likely contains hormone-disrupting chemicals (phthalates). Choose essential oils or natural perfumes instead.

Non-Stick Cookware (Teflon)

Contains PFOAs, which mess with thyroid hormones. Swap for stainless steel, ceramic, or cast iron pans.

Processed Sugar & Artificial Sweeteners

Sugar spikes insulin and inflammation, while fake sweeteners confuse your metabolism. Go for raw honey, maple syrup, or coconut sugar instead.

Tap Water

Contains chlorine, fluoride, and heavy metals that disrupt hormones. Get a high-quality water filter to protect your system.

Detoxing Through Movement

You don't have to run a marathon (unless you want to), but movement is key for detox. Your lymphatic system, which flushes toxins out of your body, doesn't have a pump—it only moves when you do.

Best Workouts for Detox:

Walking
The simplest, most underrated way to boost circulation and lymph flow.

Yoga & Stretching
Twists and deep breathing stimulate digestion and detox pathways.

Strength Training
Builds muscle, boosts metabolism, and supports hormone balance.

Rebounding (Mini Trampoline Workouts)
Literally the best thing for lymphatic drainage—plus, it's super fun.

Infrared Sauna or Epsom Salt Baths
Sweating is one of the best ways to eliminate toxins (plus, it's relaxing as hell).

Poop, Pee, & Periods

Yes, *this* is detox too—and it's essential. If you're not eliminating waste properly, you're not detoxing.

Pooping
Your liver dumps used-up hormones, toxins, and waste into your digestive tract. If you're constipated, those excess hormones get reabsorbed (yikes).

Peeing
Your kidneys flush toxins out of your system—so drink up!

Your Period
Your cycle is a natural hormone reset. If your periods are too heavy, irregular, or painful, it could be a sign your detox pathways need support.

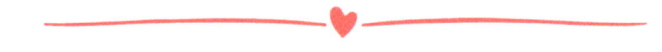

Detox isn't about deprivation. It's about devotion.
It's not punishment for what you've eaten. It's a ritual of reconnection – with your body, your energy, and your balance. When you support your detox pathways, you support your hormones. And when your hormones are happy, *you* are powerful.

So skip the trends. Burn the cleanse flyers. And remember: your body doesn't need a reboot. It needs room to do what it already knows how to do.

Let it release. Let it restore. Let it return to you.

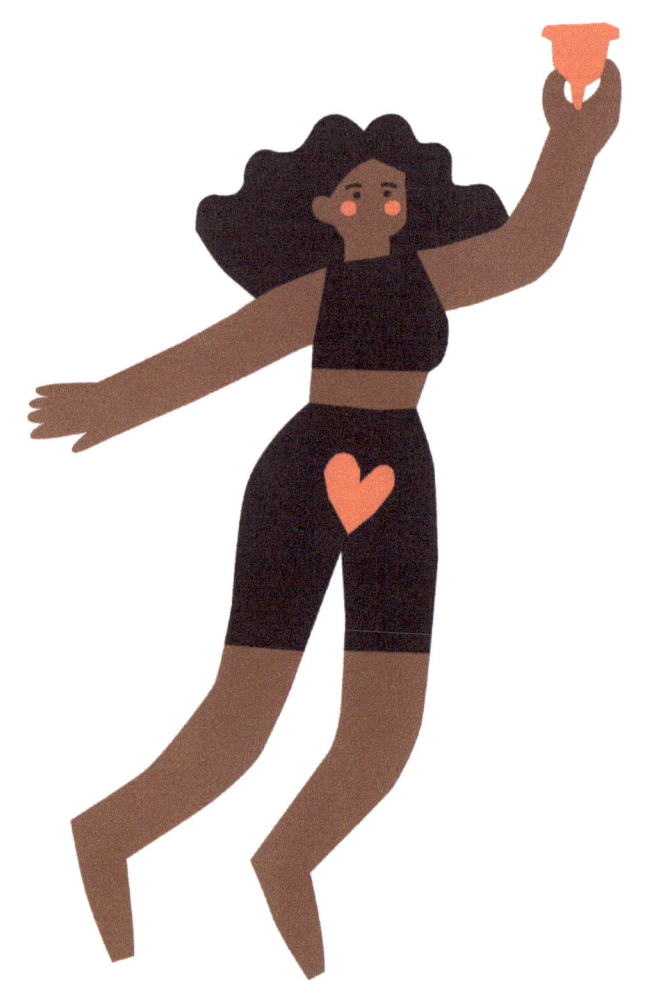

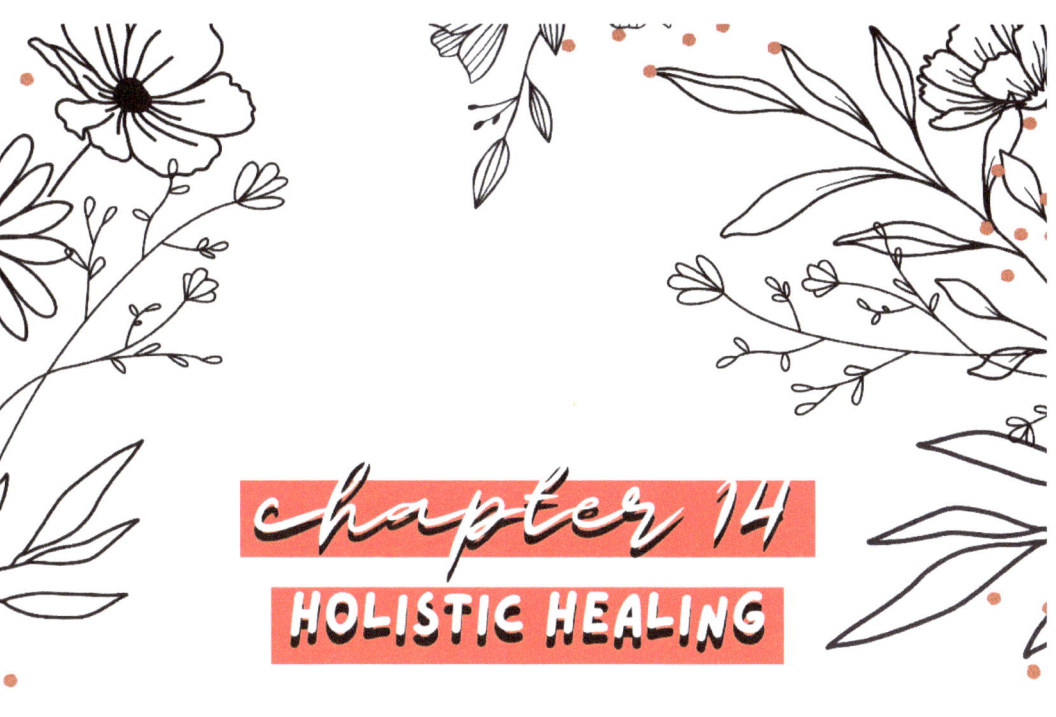

Chapter 14
Holistic Healing

Modern medicine has its place. It's saved lives, eased pain, and given us access to tools our great-grandmothers could only dream of. But sometimes the "solutions" we're handed feel like temporary patches, not true healing. Another prescription. Another shrug. Another "it's normal" when your gut, womb, or spirit says otherwise.

Enter holistic healing modalities. Ancient wisdom meets modern wellness. These practices aren't just "woo-woo hippie magic"—they're time-tested methods passed down by midwives, herbalists, grandmothers, and healers who *listened* to the body instead of silencing it.

Let's walk through some of the most powerful modalities for hormonal and reproductive healing. You don't have to try them all. Just start with what resonates, and let your intuition lead the way.

Acupuncture

Acupuncture might look like something out of a medieval sketchbook, but it's one of the most effective, science-backed tools for hormonal health.

The Reason It Works:

- Increases blood flow to the ovaries and uterus
- Balances stress and reproductive hormones
- Reduces PMS, cramps, bloating, and irritability
- Lowers inflammation and improves egg quality

Book a session with an acupuncturist who specializes in reproductive wellness. Even once a week can make a difference. Pair your appointment with breathwork, a cozy nap, or a cup of ginger or raspberry leaf tea to amplify the benefits.

Ayurveda

Ayurveda is more than golden milk and dosha quizzes. It's a 5,000-year-old system of aligning your health with the rhythms of nature – using food, herbs, oil, breath, and intuition to bring balance where there's chaos.

The Reason It Works:

- Balances estrogen and progesterone through food and herbs

- Reduces stress (and cortisol) by syncing with your body's natural cycles

- Supports digestion and detox – essential for hormonal harmony

- Regulates periods with grounding, womb-nourishing practices

Eat cycle-supportive meals—warm, cooked foods during your luteal and menstrual phases; light, cooling foods in the follicular and ovulatory phases.

Practice Abhyanga, a warm oil self-massage using sesame or coconut oil to ground your nervous system and soothe cramps. Explore Ayurvedic herbs like shatavari (balances estrogen and supports fertility) and ashwagandha (lowers cortisol and boosts libido).

Yoni Steaming

Yoni steaming is an ancient practice with roots in African, Indigenous, and Asian healing systems, and it's making a powerful comeback. This isn't just a vaginal "cleanse." It's a ritual of restoration. A way to connect with your womb, release stuck energy, and invite healing into the pelvic bowl.

The Reason It Works:

- Increases circulation to the uterus and vaginal tissues

- Reduces cramps, clotting, and heavy bleeding

- Supports postpartum healing and minimizes old residue from past cycles
  • Deepens connection to your womb space and feminine energy

Steam 1-2 times per cycle using herbs like mugwort, rosemary, lavender, and red raspberry leaf. Never steam while menstruating or if pregnant, and be cautious if you have an IUD. Pair your steam with deep breathing, journaling, or womb massage for a deeper release.

Herbal Medicine

Herbs aren't "alternative." They're original. Before pharmaceuticals, women healed with roots, leaves, and flowers that knew exactly how to speak to the body.

Vitex (Chasteberry)
Boosts progesterone, supports ovulation, and helps regulate cycles

Red Raspberry Leaf
Tones the uterus and supports balanced periods

Nettle & Dandelion - Help your liver clear excess estrogen (which is often the root of PMS and heavy bleeding)

Brew herbal teas during your luteal or menstrual phases. Add herbs to your castor oil packs for a deeper detox. Use tinctures or capsules for consistency if tea isn't your thing. Herbs work slowly and deeply. Let them build trust with your body.

Medicinal Mushrooms

Functional mushrooms like Reishi, Cordyceps, and Lion's Mane aren't just for your smoothie. They're powerful adaptogens. They help the body adapt to stress and return to balance.

- **Reishi –** The mushroom of calm. Lowers cortisol and helps you sleep.

- **Cordyceps** – Boosts libido, stamina, and energy.

- **Lion's Mane –** Brain and mood support, especially during hormonal transitions like postpartum or perimenopause.

Try them in tea, tinctures, or capsules. Just make sure they're organic and from a trusted source.

Castor Oil Packs

Castor oil packs are a simple, ancient remedy that support detox, hormone regulation, and pelvic health – and they feel like a mini spa treatment.

Why it works:

- Increases circulation to the uterus and ovaries
- Supports lymphatic drainage (goodbye bloating and stagnation)
- Eases cramps and reduce painful, heavy, or
- irregular periods

How to do it:

1. Soak a soft flannel or cloth in organic castor oil
2. Place over your lower belly
3. Cover with a towel and heating pad
4. Relax for 30-45 minutes while you read, journal, or rest

Do this a few times a week, especially during your luteal phase or between periods.

Building Your Holistic Routine

Holistic care isn't about doing *everything*. It's about tuning in and creating rituals that feel nurturing – not overwhelming.

Here's a gentle starter flow:

Morning
Herbal tea, sunlight on your skin, light movement

Afternoon
Nourishing food, breathwork or walking

Evening
Castor oil pack, magnesium, yoni steam or oil massage

Weekly reset
Rebounding, sauna, or deep journaling session

And above all? Rest. Honor your body's rhythm. Holistic care starts with listening.

Modern medicine can be powerful. But healing – deep, cyclical, soul-level healing – often begins in the rituals passed down, the herbs your grandmother swore by, the quiet trust between your body and the earth.

These holistic tools aren't fads. They're ancestral. And when used with care, they invite you back into harmony – not just with your hormones, but with yourself.

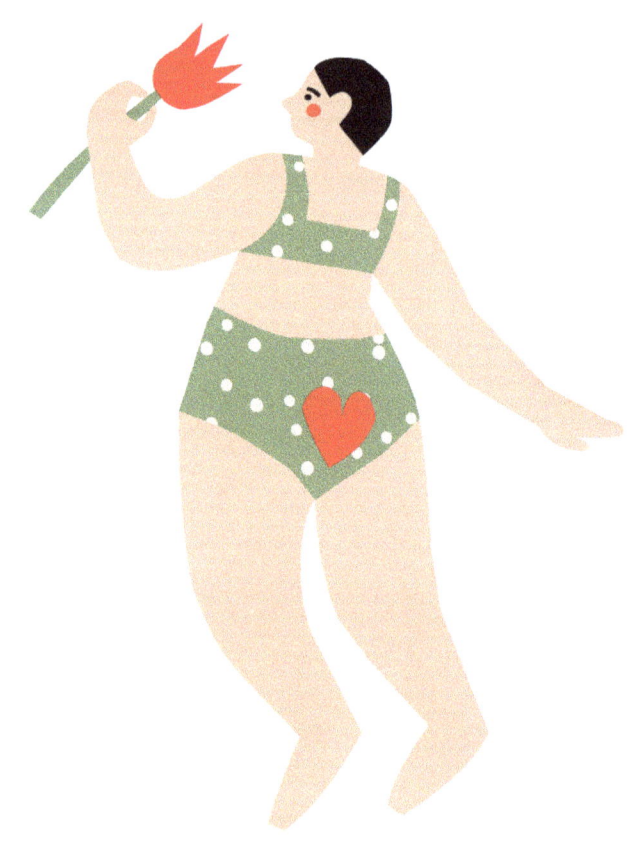

Chapter 15
THE ALCHEMY OF HER

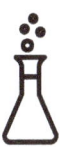

You made it, love. We've traveled through every twist and turn of womanhood—hormones, periods, gut health, infections, stress, libido, and everything in between. You've learned how your body works, what it needs, and how to care for it with intention. But before you close this book, there's one last thing I need you to remember: You are powerful.

Your Body, Your Story

This isn't just about having balanced hormones, glowing skin, or a cycle that runs like clockwork. This is about reclaiming your health, your body, and your power—on your terms.

Your body isn't just a machine—it's a masterpiece in motion. From puberty to menopause, from fertility to libido, it constantly shifts, adapts, and carries you through every stage of life. And yet, we're often taught to fight it, to see it as something that needs to be "fixed" rather than something to be honored.

Your period isn't a burden; it's a vital sign. It tells you what's going on inside, and learning to track it gives you insight into your overall health.

Your gut isn't just about digestion; it's your second brain. Taking care of it means taking care of your hormones, skin, mood, and metabolism.

Your stress levels affect everything. Learning to slow down and prioritize yourself isn't indulgent—it's essential.

Your body changes, and that's normal. Puberty, pregnancy, postpartum, menopause—your body isn't meant to stay the same forever. Learn to work with it, not against it.

Loving your body doesn't mean loving every single part of it every single day. It means respecting it, listening to it, and giving it what it needs.

The Common Threads

I know, I know. No matter what we talked about—libido, acne, fatigue, or cramps—some truths kept showing up.
You were probably like, "Here we go again…" or *"Wait… didn't she say this already?"* And yes. Yes, I did. Multiple times. On purpose. Because when something shows up in every single chapter – from PMS to libido to random chin hairs – it's not a coincidence. It's a flashing neon sign from your body saying: *"Hey girl, do this stuff."* So, without further ado, let's recap on The Foundations of Her.

- Hydrate deeply. Water + minerals = energy, digestion, and hormone flow.

- Sleep like it's sacred—because it is. Your hormones repair while you rest.

- Eat whole, vibrant foods. What you eat is information for your body.
- Move with love, not punishment. Build strength, honor rest, feel joy.

- Manage stress, don't normalize it. Cortisol can't be ignored. Breathe. Walk. Say no.
- Eliminate daily. Poop, sweat, bleed. That's how your body releases what it no longer needs.

- Get outside. Sunlight anchors your rhythms. Fresh air renews your nervous system.

- Listen inward. Symptoms are your body's way of asking for help. Start tuning in.

It's not about doing everything perfectly, it's about doing the things that matter consistently. These are your tools. Your rhythm. Your blueprint.

At the end of the day, hormone balance isn't about quick fixes. It's about small, consistent habits that support your body's natural rhythms. Master these, and you're not just surviving, you're thriving

You Are Your Own Best Healer

One of the biggest takeaways from this journey? You are the expert on your body.
Yes, doctors, nutritionists, and wellness practitioners can offer valuable guidance, but no one lives in your body but you. If something feels off, don't ignore it. If you're not getting the answers you need, keep asking. If a treatment plan doesn't sit right with you, explore alternatives.

Trust your instincts.
If a doctor dismisses your concerns or tells you something is "just part of being a woman," push back. Get a second opinion if necessary.

Do your own research.

Not all information is created equal, but learning about your body empowers you to make informed decisions.

Know your options.
From conventional medicine to holistic remedies, the best approach is the one that works for you.

Your health is not a one-size-fits-all situation. Be your own advocate, ask questions, and never settle for feeling less than your best.

This book isn't just about wellness; it's about alchemy—the transformation of knowledge into action, of care into confidence, of womanhood into power.

You now know what your body needs to thrive. The question is: will you give yourself permission to step into that power?

Because when women are healthy, balanced, and thriving, we don't just change our own lives. We change the world.

So go on. Take what you've learned, listen to your body, and step into the most radiant, empowered version of yourself.

You've got this

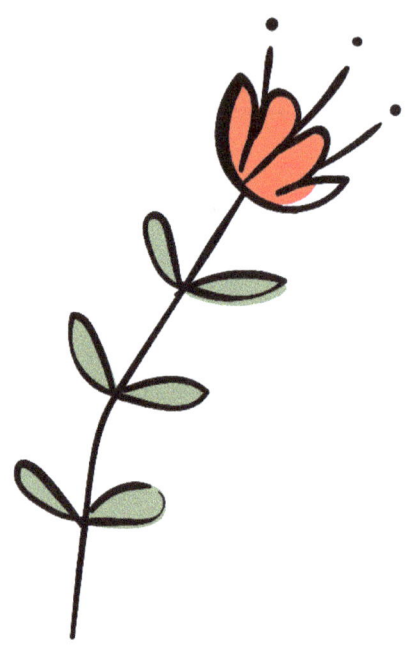

She has walked through fire and emerged gold, turning every loss into knowing, every scar into strength. No longer becoming, she simply is. The work is complete, her transformation fulfilled— alchemy realized. In her presence, the world cannot deny her magic, and the future bends to meet her.

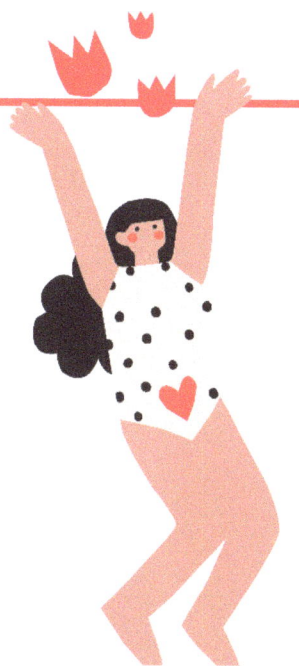

THE SECRET FORMULAS *to her* ALCHEMY

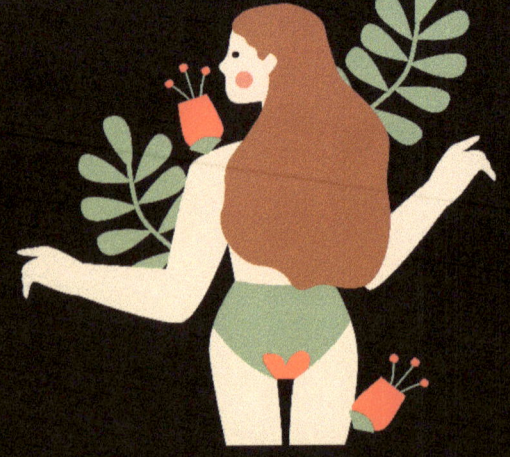

THE *bonus pages*

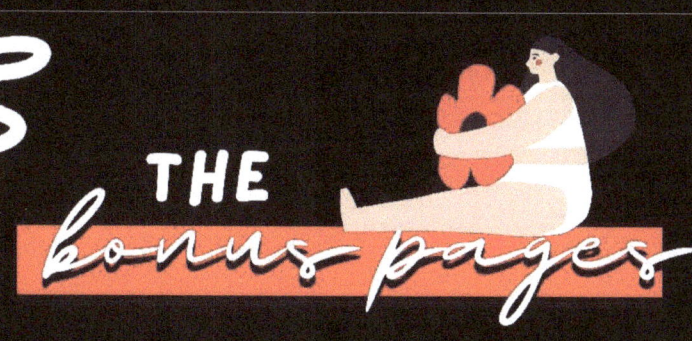

01	THE LAWS OF HER	210
02	HOW TO CLEAN HER	212
03	HER WELNESS CHECKLIST	214
04	HER HORMONES	216
05	HER DECADES	222
06	HER GLOSSARY	227
07	HER GROCERY LIST	231
08	HER RESOURCES	237
09	HER NOTES	238
10	ABOUT THE AUTHOR	244
11	SOURCES & CITATIONS	247

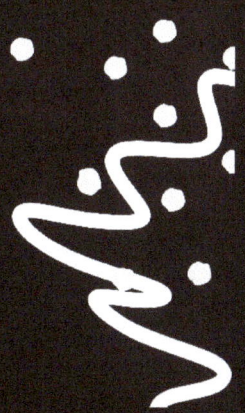
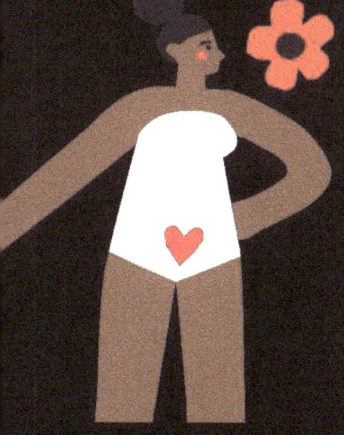

THE LAWS OF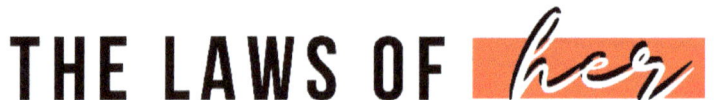

1) **GET YOUR ANNUAL CHECK-UP**
   NOT JUST A SUGGESTION

2) **ALWAYS WIPE FRONT TO BACK**
   BECAUSE UTIS ARE NOT THE VIBE

3) **KEGELS, BABE**
   YOUR PELVIC FLOOR WILL THANK YOU

4) **HYDRATION**
   FLUSH OUT THE BAD

5) **LET HER BREATHE**
   COMMANDO FOR THE WIN

6) **PH-FRIENDLY ONLY**
   USE GENTAL, MICROBIOME FRIENDLY PRODUCTS

7) **TAKE YOUR PROBIOTICS**
   ESPECIALLY AFTER ANTIBIOTICS

8) **FUEL UP ON PREBIOTICS**
   GARLIC, ONIONS, BANANAS, FLAXSEEDS...

9) **YOUR PARTNER'S HYGIENE MATTERS**
   A CLEAN MOUTH, CLEAN HANDS, CLEAN... EVERYTHING ELSE

THE LAWS OF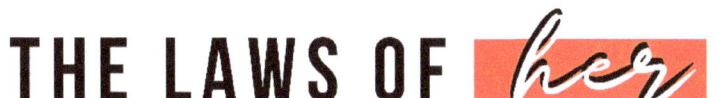

10) *LISTEN TO YOUR BODY*
    PAIN, WEIRD DISCHARGE, FUNKY SMELLS? DON'T IGNORE HER!

11) *MAKE SELFCARE NON-NEGOTIABLE*
    REST, MOVE, NOURISH, AND PROTECT YOUR PEACE

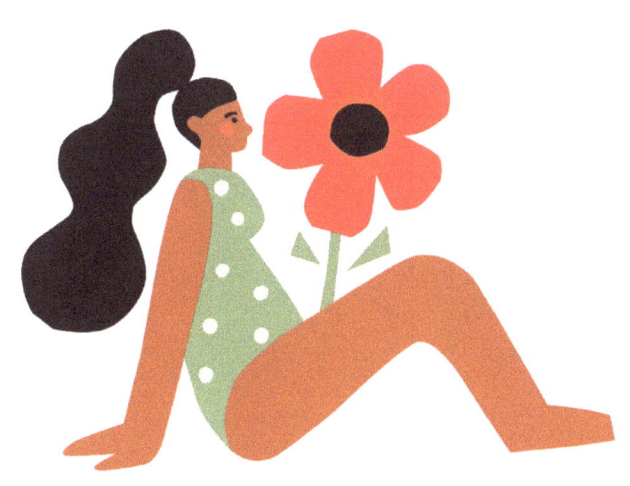

HOW TO CLEAN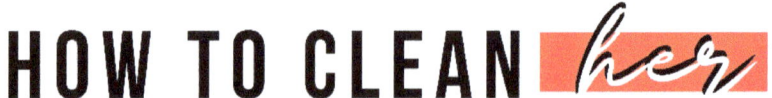

Your vagina is self-cleaning. She doesn't need soap. She doesn't need scents. She doesn't need you reaching up there with a squeeze bottle or scrubbing like you're trying to clean a bathtub.

But your vulva and other parts— that's skin. And like any other part of your body, she deserves to be kept clean gently and with respect.

Keep it simple. Here's how:

- Use warm water and your hand or a soft cloth to gently rinse the vulva. That's it.
- If you want to use soap, make sure it's mild, unscented, and only for the outside.
- Never put soap *inside* the vagina. She's got her own system.
- Wipe front to back, always. Keeps bacteria away from where it doesn't belong.
- Use a separate washcloth for your butt. Just trust me.
- Feel free to strike Pose 28 in the shower if it helps you get a better angle. You're not alone.

HOW TO CLEAN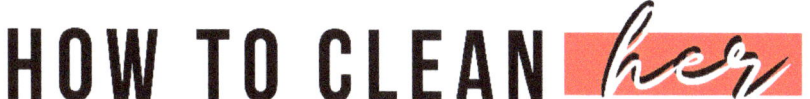

What not to do:

- No douching. Ever. It messes up your pH and leaves you more prone to infections.

- No heavily fragranced soaps, sprays, or wipes. If it smells like a tropical fruit basket, it probably doesn't belong down there.

- Don't scrub. Your vulva isn't dirty—it's delicate.

Little extras (if you want to go the extra mile):

- Let her breathe sometimes. Cotton undies or no undies to bed can help prevent sweat and irritation.

- Stay hydrated and eat clean. Your vagina reflects what's happening inside your body.

- A daily probiotic can support your vaginal flora and keep things balanced.

her WELLNESS CHECKLIST

🌸 ROUTINE SCREENINGS

- **PAP SMEAR** – EVERY 3 YEARS (AGES 21-65)

- **HPV TEST** – EVERY 5 YEARS (AGE 30+) OR WITH ABNORMAL PAP RESULTS

- **MAMMOGRAM** – EVERY 1-2 YEARS (STARTING AT AGE 40, OR EARLIER IF HIGH RISK)

- **BLOOD PRESSURE & CHOLESTEROL** – ANNUALLY OR AS RECOMMENDED

- **BLOOD SUGAR / A1C TEST** – ESPECIALLY IF OVER 45, PREGNANT, OR AT RISK

- **THYROID CHECK** – ESPECIALLY POSTPARTUM OR IF EXPERIENCING FATIGUE, WEIGHT CHANGES, OR MOOD SHIFTS

🌸 HORMONE & REPRODUCTIVE HEALTH

- **CYCLE TRACKING** - MONITOR PATTERNS, OVULATION, AND SYMPTOMS MONTHLY

- **PELVIC FLOOR HEALTH** - WATCH FOR SIGNS LIKE LEAKAGE, HEAVINESS, OR PAIN

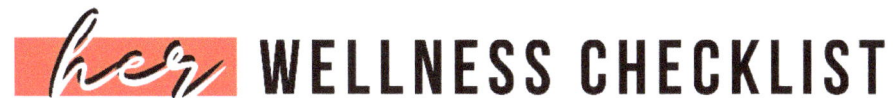 WELLNESS CHECKLIST

- **BREAST SELF-EXAM** – MONTHLY CHECK FOR LUMPS, CHANGES, OR PAIN

- **FERTILITY AWARENESS** – KNOW YOUR BODY'S RHYTHMS WHETHER YOU'RE CONCEIVING OR NOT

 OPTIONAL LAB PANELS TO CONSIDER

- FULL HORMONE PANEL (ESTROGEN, PROGESTERONE, TESTOSTERONE, CORTISOL)

- VITAMIN D & B12

- IRON & FERRITIN

- INFLAMMATORY MARKERS (CRP, ESR)

- COMPREHENSIVE METABOLIC PANEL

- GENETIC SCREENING IF PLANNING PREGNANCY OR MANAGING HEALTH RISKS

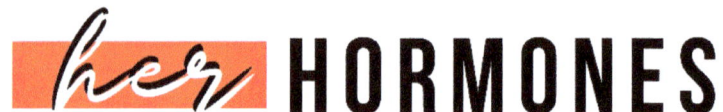 # HORMONES

ESTROGEN
"The Glow-Up Queen"

This is the hormone that gives you curves, mood swings, and that dewy skin glow when she's feeling generous.
- Helps regulate your menstrual cycle
- Supports skin, bones, and brain function
- Drops during menopause, which can lead to hot flashes, dry skin, and irritability

---

PROGESTERONE
"The Chill Pill"

She keeps things calm, cozy, and balanced—especially after ovulation.
- Prepares the uterus for pregnancy
- Supports deeper sleep and reduces anxiety
- Low levels can mean PMS, restlessness, and mood shifts

TESTOSTERONE
"The Silent Powerhouse"

Often thought of as the "male hormone," but women need it too—for energy, drive, and muscle tone.
- Fuels libido and motivation
- Helps build strength and confidence

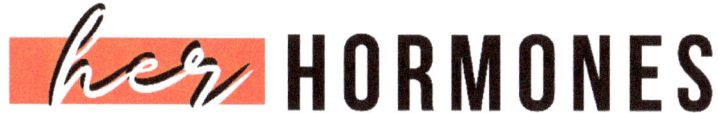 **HORMONES**

- Too much? Think PCOS, acne, and facial hair

PROLACTIN
"Milk Mama"

She's all about nurturing. High after childbirth, she supports milk production and that mama-baby bond.
- Stimulates breast milk
- Helps calm the nervous system post-birth
- Can delay ovulation while breastfeeding

OXYTOCIN
"The Connection Hormone"

Released when you hug, kiss, orgasm, give birth, or even make strong eye contact.
- Encourages bonding and trust
- Plays a role in labor contractions and milk letdown
- Helps regulate emotional closeness

FSH (FOLLICLE-STIMULATING HORMONE)
"Egg Coach"

This one rallies the follicles in your ovaries to grow and mature.
- Key to getting ovulation started
- Helps balance your cycle
- Works closely with estrogen and LH

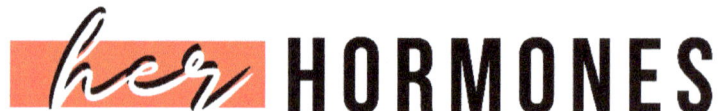# HORMONES

LH (LUTEINIZING HORMONE)
"The Ovulation Trigger"

LH surges mid-cycle to release an egg from the ovary.
- Responsible for ovulation
- Essential for fertility
- Works alongside FSH like a hormonal tag team

GNRH (GONADOTROPIN-RELEASING HORMONE)
"The Brain Signal"

Released from the hypothalamus in the brain, this one cues the body to begin the monthly hormone process.
- Tells the pituitary to release FSH and LH
- Keeps your reproductive cycle in motion
- Starts up during puberty and runs the whole show from there

---

HCG (HUMAN CHORIONIC GONADOTROPIN)
"The Pregnancy Signal"

If fertilization happens, this hormone is what keeps the pregnancy stable in early weeks.
- Detected in pregnancy tests
- Helps maintain high progesterone in early pregnancy
- Supports the uterine lining so baby can stay snug

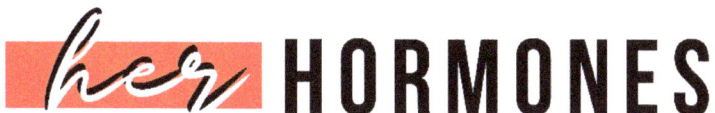# her HORMONES

CORTISOL
"The Stress Responder"

This hormone isn't all bad—it wakes you up in the morning and gets you through tough moments. But too much for too long? That's when it causes chaos.
- Helps regulate blood sugar, energy, and inflammation
- Supports the body during stress
- Chronic elevation = weight gain, anxiety, period issues, burnout

INSULIN
"The Sugar Balancer"

She's in charge of helping your cells use sugar for energy. But when she's overworked, she can throw everything off.
- Regulates blood sugar levels
- Affects hunger, cravings, and fat storage
- Imbalances are linked to fatigue, PCOS, and insulin resistance

MELATONIN
"The Sleep Regulator"

She follows your circadian rhythm and helps you wind down at night.
- Rises in the evening to make you sleepy
- Drops in the morning with sunlight

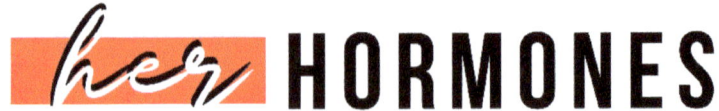

her HORMONES

- Disrupted by screens, stress, or irregular sleep patterns

THYROID HORMONES (T3, T4)
"The Metabolism Monitors"

These hormones regulate how fast your body uses energy—and they impact everything from mood to digestion.
- Support metabolism, heart rate, and menstrual cycles
- Low thyroid = fatigue, weight gain, brain fog
- High thyroid = anxiety, rapid heartbeat, trouble sleeping

DOPAMINE
"The Motivation Spark"

This one helps you feel pleasure, focus, and drive. When dopamine's low, everything feels harder.
- Supports productivity and reward
- Linked to focus, attention, and willpower
- Boosted by movement, sleep, and joyful experiences

SEROTONIN
"The Mood Stabilizer"

About 90% of this feel-good hormone is actually made in your gut.
- Supports emotional regulation
- Affects sleep, digestion, and appetite

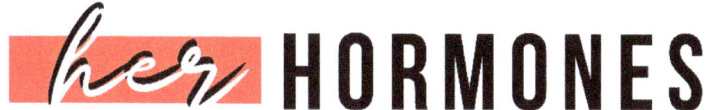 # HORMONES

- Balanced by sunlight, gut health, and calming routines

ENDORPHINS
"The Natural Painkillers"

Released when you exercise, laugh, cry, or climax—they help you feel better when life hurts.
- Reduce pain naturally
- Boost mood and mental clarity
- Triggered by movement, joy, and deep connection

DHEA
"The Hormone Precursor"

It's like the raw material your body uses to make estrogen and testosterone.
- Supports energy, libido, and hormonal balance
- Peaks in your 20s and slowly declines
- Healthy fats and strength training can help maintain levels

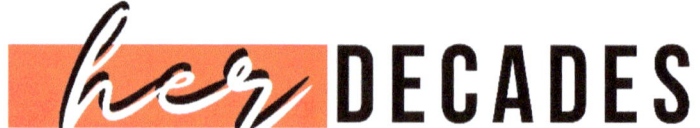
her DECADES

🌸 TEENS (13-19)

- Begin tracking your cycle to learn your body's rhythm.

- Eat nourishing foods that support brain, skin, and hormone health.

- Establish a healthy relationship with your body—free of shame.

- Talk openly about periods, consent, and pleasure-positive education.

- Introduce gentle movement (dance, walking, yoga) as a lifestyle.

- Learn about vaginal care, hygiene, and how to protect your microbiome.

- Prioritize sleep—it's foundational for growth and emotional regulation.

🌸 TWENTIES

- Schedule your first pap smear, sti test, and annual wellness visits.

- Start supplementing with vitamin d, omega-3s, and iron if needed.

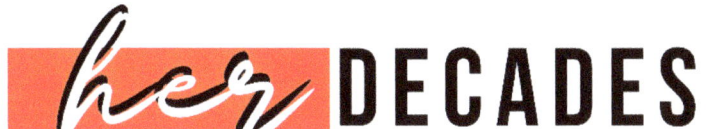
DECADES

- Stay consistent with movement—muscle memory starts now.

- Focus on gut health (hello probiotics, fiber, and fermented foods).

- Build a sacred self-care practice: rest, journaling, breathwork.

- Learn the language of your libido—what turns you on and why it matters..

❀ THIRTIES

- Get proactive with hormone health (test estrogen, thyroid, etc).

- Rebalance after birth control, postpartum, or fertility challenges.

- Strength train to protect bones and shape your curves.

- Fuel your nervous system with magnesium, adaptogens, and healthy fats.

- Honor emotional shifts—this decade often brings identity evolution.

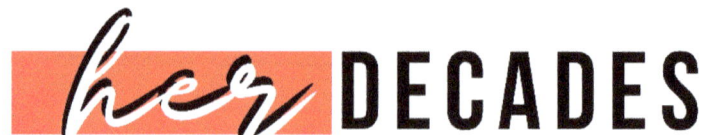

- Consider fertility mapping or preservation if desired for future family planning.

🌸 FORTIES

- Get your mammogram and full labs (hormones, thyroid, cholesterol, A1C).

- Embrace perimenopause: track symptoms, nourish adrenal glands, reduce caffeine.

- Prioritize heart health, libido, and stress resilience.

- Address mood swings or cycle changes early—your body is talking.

- Release what no longer serves—this is a decade of transformation.

- Learn pelvic floor exercises and vaginal dryness solutions proactively.

🌸 FIFTIES

- Menopause may arrive—learn your hormone levels and options (HRT, herbs, lifestyle).

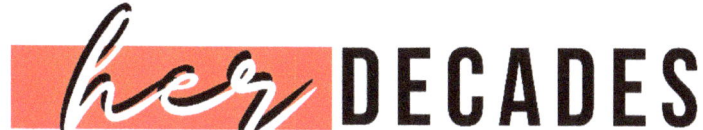
her DECADES

- Balance blood sugar, weight, and bone density with protein, strength training, and minerals.

- Get screened for colon cancer, diabetes, and osteoporosis.

- Reclaim pleasure—vaginal care and sexual health don't expire.

- Prioritize rest, mental health, and joy over hustle culture.

- Explore legacy-building: writing, teaching, nurturing community.

🌸 SIXTIES

- Protect cognitive function with omega-3s, puzzles, new learning, and social connection.

- Stay active (yoga, walking, swimming) to keep joints and heart strong.

- Address bladder health, prolapse, or thinning vaginal tissue gently.
- Reframe aging as an initiation, not a decline—your wisdom blooms here.

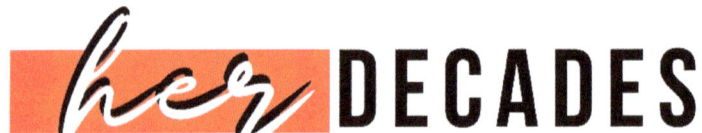

her DECADES

- Get annual exams: mammogram, cholesterol, bone scan, etc.

- Prioritize rest, mental health, and joy over hustle culture.

- Explore legacy-building: writing, teaching, nurturing community.

❁ SEVENTIES & WISER

- Prioritize fall prevention, bone health, and hydration.

- Keep moving: tai chi, resistance bands, gardening, dancing.

- Speak up about sleep, sex, or digestion concerns—nothing is "just age."

- Connect deeply—relationships and purpose keep the soul alive.

- Continue wellness checks and stay current with vaccines.

- Celebrate your life force—your presence is medicine.

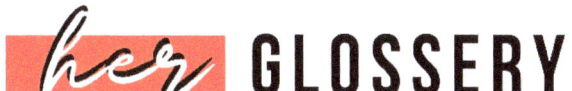 **GLOSSERY**

 HERBS & BOTINCALS

ASHWAGANDHA - LOWERS CORTISOL (STRESS HORMONE), IMPROVES SLEEP, REDUCES ANXIETY, AND HELPS WITH HORMONAL BALANCE.

DANDELION ROOT - SUPPORTS LIVER DETOX, REDUCES WATER RETENTION & BLOATING, HELPS ELIMINATE EXCESS ESTROGEN.

HOLY BASIL (TULSI) - LOWERS STRESS & ANXIETY, SUPPORTS BLOOD SUGAR BALANCE & DIGESTION.

GINGER & TURMERIC - REDUCE INFLAMMATION, SUPPORT DIGESTION & DETOX, HELP WITH PAIN & CRAMPS.

NETTLE LEAF - NUTRIENT-DENSE HERB RICH IN IRON & MINERALS, SUPPORTS HORMONAL BALANCE, REDUCES INFLAMMATION.

MACA ROOT - BOOSTS LIBIDO, ENERGY, AND MOOD, SUPPORTS FERTILITY, AND BALANCES ESTROGEN & TESTOSTERONE.

MILK THISTLE - PROTECTS & REGENERATES THE LIVER, CLEARS OUT HORMONE-DISRUPTING TOXINS, SUPPORTS SKIN HEALTH.

RED RASPBERRY LEAF - STRENGTHENS THE UTERUS, SUPPORTS MENSTRUAL HEALTH & FERTILITY, REDUCES CRAMPING.

RHODIOLA - REDUCES BURNOUT & FATIGUE, BOOSTS MENTAL CLARITY & ENERGY, SUPPORTS ADRENAL HEALTH.

SPEARMINT TEA - REDUCES TESTOSTERONE LEVELS (GREAT FOR PCOS ACNE & EXCESS HAIR GROWTH), SUPPORTS HORMONAL BALANCE.

VITEX (CHASTE TREE BERRY) - SUPPORTS PROGESTERONE PRODUCTION, HELPS REGULATE CYCLES, REDUCES PMS & LUTEAL PHASE ISSUES.

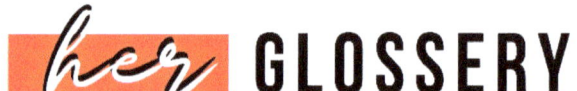 # GLOSSERY

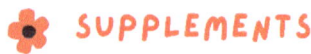 ## SUPPLEMENTS

ADAPTOGENIC MUSHROOM BLENDS (REISHI, CORDYCEPS, LION'S MANE) - REDUCE STRESS & INFLAMMATION, IMPROVE ENERGY & FOCUS, SUPPORT HORMONAL HEALTH.

B-COMPLEX VITAMINS - HELPS WITH ENERGY, MOOD, METABOLISM, SUPPORTS DETOX PATHWAYS.

COLLAGEN PEPTIDES - STRENGTHENS HAIR, SKIN, NAILS, & GUT LINING, SUPPORTS JOINT HEALTH.

INOSITOL (MYO- & D-CHIRO) - ESSENTIAL FOR PCOS, IMPROVES INSULIN SENSITIVITY, SUPPORTS OVULATION & CYCLE REGULATION.

IRON (WITH VITAMIN C) - PREVENTS HAIR LOSS, FATIGUE, & HEAVY PERIODS, ESPECIALLY IMPORTANT FOR THOSE WITH LOW FERRITIN.

MAGNESIUM CITRATE - HELPS WITH DIGESTION & CONSTIPATION, SUPPORTS GUT HEALTH.

MAGNESIUM GLYCINATE - SUPPORTS RELAXATION, DEEP SLEEP, STRESS REDUCTION, HELPS WITH PMS & MUSCLE TENSION.

OMEGA-3S (FISH OIL OR FLAXSEED OIL) - REDUCES INFLAMMATION, BALANCES HORMONES, IMPROVES SKIN & BRAIN HEALTH.

PROBIOTICS - SUPPORTS GUT HEALTH, CLEARS SKIN, IMPROVES DIGESTION, HELPS WITH HORMONAL DETOX.

SELENIUM & IODINE - CRUCIAL FOR THYROID HEALTH, IMPROVES METABOLISM & HORMONE PRODUCTION.

VITAMIN D3 + K2 - SUPPORTS IMMUNE HEALTH, MOOD, BONE STRENGTH, HELPS WITH HORMONE BALANCE.

ZINC - BOOSTS IMMUNE FUNCTION, REDUCES ACNE, SUPPORTS TESTOSTERONE BALANCE & FERTILITY.

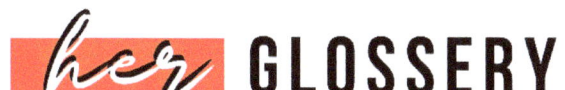

her GLOSSERY

❋ EXERCISE AND MOVEMENT

DANCE & CARDIO (IN MODERATION!) - HELPS BLOOD CIRCULATION & ENERGY, BUT AVOID EXCESSIVE CARDIO IF STRESSED OR DEALING WITH ADRENAL FATIGUE.

PELVIC FLOOR EXERCISES (KEGELS & RELAXATION) - IMPROVES SENSATION, BLADDER CONTROL, AND SUPPORTS HEALTHY SEXUAL FUNCTION.

REBOUNDING (MINI TRAMPOLINE WORKOUTS) - BEST EXERCISE FOR LYMPHATIC DRAINAGE, SUPPORTS DETOX & IMMUNE SYSTEM.

STRENGTH TRAINING - PREVENTS MUSCLE LOSS, SUPPORTS METABOLISM, BALANCES BLOOD SUGAR, BOOSTS TESTOSTERONE & GROWTH HORMONE.

WALKING - BEST LOW-IMPACT EXERCISE FOR HORMONAL BALANCE, STRESS REDUCTION, DIGESTION, & LYMPHATIC FLOW.

YOGA & STRETCHING - SUPPORTS STRESS RELIEF, PELVIC FLOOR STRENGTH, PERIOD PAIN RELIEF, AND HORMONE BALANCE.

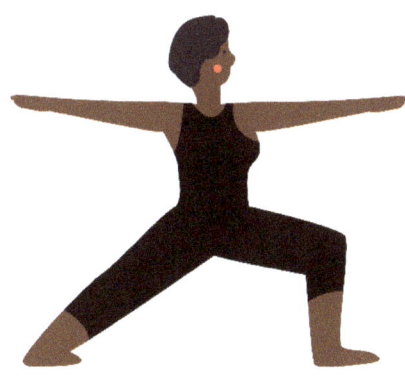

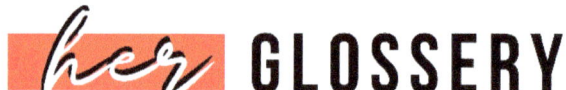 # GLOSSERY

🌸 HOLISTIC PRACTICES

ACUPUNCTURE - AN ANCIENT CHINESE HEALING PRACTICE THAT STIMULATES ENERGY FLOW THROUGH SPECIFIC POINTS IN THE BODY. HELPS REGULATE HORMONES, REDUCE STRESS, SUPPORT FERTILITY, RELIEVE PAIN, AND RESTORE NERVOUS SYSTEM BALANCE.

AYURVEDA (THE SCIENCE OF LIFE) - A HOLISTIC HEALING SYSTEM FROM INDIA THAT BALANCES THE BODY THROUGH PERSONALIZED FOOD, HERBS, LIFESTYLE, AND SELF-CARE RITUALS BASED ON YOUR DOSHA (MIND-BODY TYPE). SUPPORTS DIGESTION, HORMONE BALANCE, AND CYCLE HEALTH.

CASTOR OIL PACKS (ON ABDOMEN) - SUPPORTS LIVER DETOX, DIGESTION, HORMONE BALANCE, FERTILITY, AND PERIOD HEALTH.

CYCLE SYNCING (EATING & EXERCISING ACCORDING TO YOUR CYCLE) - SUPPORTS HORMONAL BALANCE, REDUCES PMS, BOOSTS ENERGY & METABOLISM.

DEEP BREATHING & BREATHWORK (BOX BREATHING, DIAPHRAGMATIC BREATHING) - LOWERS CORTISOL & ANXIETY, SUPPORTS VAGUS NERVE & NERVOUS SYSTEM BALANCE.

DRY BRUSHING - STIMULATES LYMPHATIC FLOW & DETOX, IMPROVES SKIN TEXTURE & CIRCULATION.

REDUCING TOXIN EXPOSURE (SWITCHING TO CLEAN BEAUTY, NATURAL TAMPONS, & GLASS STORAGE CONTAINERS) - ELIMINATES ENDOCRINE DISRUPTORS THAT THROW OFF HORMONE BALANCE.
SAUNA & EPSOM SALT BATHS - HELPS WITH DETOX, RELAXATION, MUSCLE TENSION, PROMOTES LYMPHATIC DRAINAGE.

SUNLIGHT EXPOSURE (FIRST THING IN THE MORNING) - REGULATES CIRCADIAN RHYTHM, BALANCES CORTISOL, SUPPORTS VITAMIN D PRODUCTION.

YONI STEAMING - SUPPORTS VAGINAL HEALTH, CIRCULATION, UTERINE DETOX, MAY REDUCE CRAMPING & IRREGULAR PERIODS.

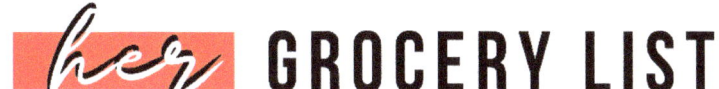 GROCERY LIST

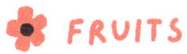 FRUITS

- **BERRIES -** PACKED WITH ANTIOXIDANTS TO BOOST BRAIN FUNCTION, PROTECT YOUR SKIN, AND SUPPORT HORMONE HEALTH.

- **BANANAS -** RICH IN POTASSIUM AND NATURAL SUGARS FOR GUT SUPPORT, MOOD BALANCE, AND CLEAN ENERGY.

- **APPLES -** A FIBER-FILLED FRIEND FOR DIGESTION AND GENTLE HORMONE DETOX.

- **CITRUS (ORANGES, LEMONS, GRAPEFRUIT) -** HIGH IN VITAMIN C TO SUPPORT IMMUNE HEALTH AND PROGESTERONE PRODUCTION.

- **POMEGRANATE -** A FERTILITY FAVORITE THAT SUPPORTS UTERINE TONE AND HEALTHY BLOOD FLOW.

- **PAPAYA -** ENZYME-RICH AND SOOTHING FOR DIGESTION, WITH ADDED PERKS FOR LACTATION AND MILK SUPPLY.

- **KIWI -** A VITAMIN C POWERHOUSE FOR RADIANT SKIN AND IMMUNE DEFENSE.

- **WATERMELON -** ULTRA-HYDRATING AND SUPPORTIVE OF KIDNEY FUNCTION AND ELECTROLYTE BALANCE.

- **DATES -** IRON-RICH AND ENERGIZING – IDEAL FOR POSTPARTUM RECOVERY AND BLOOD-BUILDING.

- **PINEAPPLE & MANGO -** ENZYME-PACKED TO REDUCE INFLAMMATION AND SPARK LIBIDO.

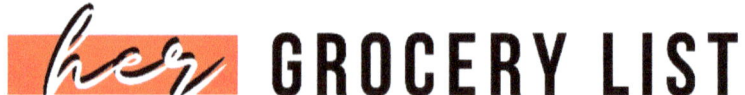 **GROCERY LIST**

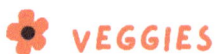 **VEGGIES**

- **BROCCOLI, CAULIFLOWER, KALE, ARUGULA** - CRUCIFEROUS QUEENS THAT HELP DETOX EXCESS ESTROGEN, SUPPORT LIVER FUNCTION, AND REBALANCE HORMONES.

- **SPINACH & SWISS CHARD -** IRON AND MAGNESIUM-RICH GREENS FOR ENERGY, MENSTRUAL SUPPORT, AND MOOD STABILIZATION.

- **SWEET POTATOES, CARROTS, BEETS –** ROOTED IN HORMONE-FRIENDLY CARBS, VITAMIN A, AND CIRCULATION-BOOSTING NUTRIENTS FOR FERTILITY AND GLOW.

- **CABBAGE & BRUSSELS SPROUTS -** GENTLE LIVER DETOXIFIERS THAT HELP EASE PMS AND SUPPORT ESTROGEN BALANCE.

- **ZUCCHINI, CUCUMBER, CELERY -** COOLING, ANTI-BLOAT STAPLES THAT AID DIGESTION AND REDUCE INFLAMMATION.

- **BELL PEPPERS & TOMATOES -** LOADED WITH ANTIOXIDANTS TO NOURISH SKIN, IMMUNITY, AND CELLULAR REPAIR.

- **ONIONS, GARLIC, LEEKS -** PREBIOTIC-RICH AND IMMUNE-BOOSTING ALLIES FOR GUT HEALTH AND MICROBIOME HARMONY.

- **SEAWEED -** A MINERAL-RICH SOURCE OF IODINE TO SUPPORT THYROID FUNCTION AND FERTILITY.

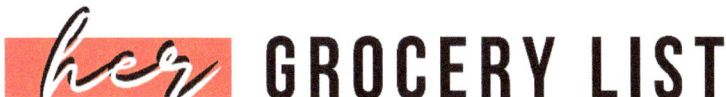 GROCERY LIST

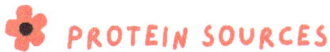 PROTEIN SOURCES

- **GRASS-FED BEEF** - A RICH SOURCE OF IRON AND ZINC TO FUEL LIBIDO, SUPPORT HORMONE PRODUCTION, AND REPLENISH YOUR BODY DURING MENSTRUATION OR POSTPARTUM.

- **PASTURE-RAISED CHICKEN** - LEAN, CLEAN PROTEIN THAT HELPS REGULATE BLOOD SUGAR AND KEEPS YOUR ENERGY STEADY ALL DAY.

- **WILD-CAUGHT SALMON** - BRIMMING WITH OMEGA-3S TO EASE INFLAMMATION, BALANCE HORMONES, AND BOOST BRAIN HEALTH.

- **ORGANIC EGGS** - PROTEIN PACKED AND LOADED WITH CHOLINE FOR FERTILITY, COGNITIVE FUNCTION, AND CELL REPAIR.

- **SARDINES & MACKEREL** - PACKED WITH CALCIUM, SELENIUM, AND ANTI-INFLAMMATORY FATS FOR BONE AND THYROID HEALTH.

PLANT BASED PROTEIN SOURCES

- **LENTILS, CHICKPEAS, BLACK BEANS, EDAMAME** - PROTEIN-PACKED AND FIBER-RICH TO SUPPORT DIGESTION, BLOOD SUGAR BALANCE, AND HORMONE HARMONY.

- **HEMP SEEDS, CHIA SEEDS, PUMPKIN SEEDS** - TINY SUPERFOODS LOADED WITH PROTEIN, OMEGA-3S, AND HORMONE-SUPPORTIVE MINERALS LIKE MAGNESIUM AND ZINC.

- **QUINOA** - A RARE PLANT-BASED COMPLETE PROTEIN THAT FUELS YOUR CYCLE, SUPPORTS YOUR MUSCLES, AND KEEPS CRAVINGS IN CHECK.

- **TEMPEH & TOFU** - FERMENTED SOY STAPLES RICH IN PHYTOESTROGENS TO GENTLY SUPPORT ESTROGEN LEVELS AND FEED YOUR GUT BACTERIA.

- **BONE BROTH OR COLLAGEN POWDER** - HEALING AND HYDRATING SUPPORT FOR GUT LINING, JOINTS, AND GLOWING SKIN – ESPECIALLY HELPFUL POSTPARTUM OR DURING HORMONAL SHIFTS.

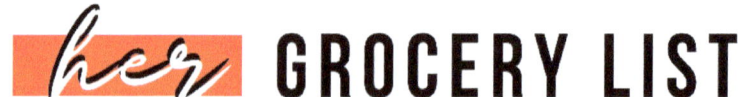

her GROCERY LIST

🌸 DAIRY

- **FULL-FAT GREEK YOGUR**T - LOADED WITH PROBIOTICS, PROTEIN, AND CALCIUM TO LOVE ON YOUR GUT, BONES, AND SKIN.

- **GRASS-FED BUTTER OR GHEE** - A RICH SOURCE OF HEALTHY FATS THAT FUEL HORMONE PRODUCTION AND HELP WITH POSTPARTUM HEALING.

- **RAW OR A2 MILK** - IF YOUR BODY AGREES, THESE TRADITIONAL FORMS OF MILK CAN BE FERTILITY-FRIENDLY AND HIGHLY NUTRIENT-DENSE.

- **GOAT CHEESE & FETA** - CREAMY, TANGY, AND OFTEN EASIER TO DIGEST THAN COW DAIRY – PLUS A GREAT SOURCE OF CALCIUM.

DAIRY ALTERNATIVES

- **COCONUT YOGURT** - CREAMY, PROBIOTIC-RICH, AND GENTLE ON YOUR GUT – PLUS SUPPORTIVE OF HORMONAL BALANCE.

- **ALMOND MILK** - LOW IN CALCIUM BUT SUPER EASY TO DIGEST; PERFECT IN SMOOTHIES, TEAS, AND HORMONE-SAFE LATTES.

- **OAT MILK** - NATURALLY COMFORTING AND A KNOWN GALACTAGOGUE (MILK-BOOSTER) – GREAT FOR MOOD AND MILK SUPPLY.

- **CASHEW MILK** - VELVETY, NUTTY, AND FILLED WITH HEALTHY FATS TO KEEP HORMONES AND SKIN NOURISHED.

- **PLANT-BASED CHEESE** (CLEAN BRANDS) - A TASTY ALT THAT SATISFIES CRAVINGS WITHOUT ADDED HORMONES OR GUT IRRITATION.

- **UNSWEETENED NUT-BASED CREAMERS** - THE GO-TO FOR CLEAN, HORMONE-FRIENDLY COFFEE AND TEA RITUALS.

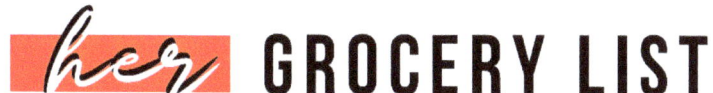 # GROCERY LIST

 ### HEALTHY FATS

- **AVOCADOS** - FOR HORMONES, SKIN, AND BRAIN SUPPORT
- **OLIVE OIL & OLIVES** - ANTI-INFLAMMATORY AND HEART-HEALTHY
- **COCONUT OIL** - ENERGY, GUT HEALTH, AND FIGHTS BAD BACTERIA
- **GHEE** - GUT-HEALING AND RICH IN FAT-SOLUBLE VITAMINS
- **GRASS-FED BUTTER** - BRAIN, MOOD, AND HORMONE HEALTH
- **NUT BUTTERS** - MINERAL-RICH, AND BLOOD SUGAR-FRIENDLY
- **BRAZIL NUTS** - SELENIUM-RICH FOR THYROID AND FERTILITY (JUST 1-2 DAILY)
- **WALNUTS** - OMEGA-3S FOR BRAIN + HORMONE SUPPORT
- **FLAXSEEDS** - BALANCES ESTROGEN AND SUPPORTS DIGESTION
- **DARK CHOCOLATE** - MAGNESIUM-RICH MOOD AND LIBIDO BOOSTER

 ### GRAINS AND CARBS

- **QUINOA** - COMPLETE PLANT PROTEIN + FIBER + BLOOD SUGAR BALANCE
- **BROWN RICE** - COMPLEX CARB FOR ENERGY AND DIGESTION
- **ROLLED OR STEEL-CUT OATS** - MILK PRODUCTION, FIBER, B VITAMINS
- **SWEET POTATOES** - HORMONE-SUPPORT, VITAMIN A, STEADY ENERGY
- **SPROUTED GRAIN BREAD** - EASIER TO DIGEST, SUPPORTS STABLE BLOOD SUGAR
- **CHICKPEA OR LENTIL PASTA** - PROTEIN + FIBER, HORMONE HEALTH
- **MILLET / AMARANTH** - DIGESTION, MINERALS, AND MILK SUPPORT
- **BUCKWHEAT** - IRON-RICH, GLUTEN-FREE, GREAT FOR CYCLE HEALTH
- **BARLEY** - TRADITIONAL MILK-BOOSTER (GALACTAGOGUE)
- **WHOLE GRAIN TORTILLAS / CRACKERS** - CONVENIENT FIBER + CARB SOURCE
- **POPCORN** (WITH COCONUT OIL) - WHOLE GRAIN + HEALTHY FATS = BLOOD SUGAR BALANCE
- **WILD RICE** - ANTIOXIDANTS + MINERAL-RICH + BLOOD SUGAR-FRIENDLY

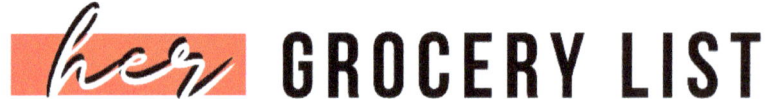 # GROCERY LIST

🌸 HYDRATION AND MINERAL SUPPORT

- FILTERED WATER
- COCONUT WATER (NATURAL ELECTROLYTES)
- HERBAL TEAS: SPEARMINT (FOR PCOS), DANDELION, NETTLE, RED RASPBERRY LEAF, TULSI
- ELECTROLYTE POWDERS OR SEA SALT + LEMON WATER
- MAGNESIUM MOCKTAILS (MAGNESIUM + MINERALS = MOOD & RELAXATION)

🌸 MINERALS AND TRACE NUTRIENTS

- HIMALAYAN PINK SALT OR SEA SALT (MINERAL-RICH)
- BRAZIL NUTS (SELENIUM = THYROID, FERTILITY)
- PUMPKIN SEEDS (ZINC = TESTOSTERONE & IMMUNE SUPPORT)
- SEAWEED / KELP FLAKES (IODINE = THYROID SUPPORT)

🌸 FUNCTIONAL ADD ONS

- CACAO NIBS OR POWDER
- GROUND FLAXSEEDS
- COLLAGEN PEPTIDES OR BONE BROTH POWDER
- HERBAL TEAS
- APPLE CIDER VINEGAR
- RAW HONEY OR MANUKA HONEY
- TAHINI (CALCIUM + HEALTHY FATS)
- COCONUT AMINOS (CLEAN SOY SAUCE ALT)
- HERBAL TINCTURES (OPTIONAL)
- MISO PASTE
- SHELF-STABLE PROBIOTIC SUPPLEMENT

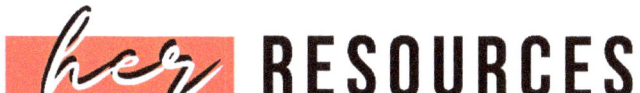 # RESOURCES

 ### MENTAL HEALTH & EMOTIONAL SUPPORT
- NATIONAL SUICIDE & CRISIS LIFELINE: 988
- SAMHSA (SUBSTANCE ABUSE & MENTAL HEALTH SERVICES): 1-800-662-HELP (4357)
- POSTPARTUM SUPPORT INTERNATIONAL (FOR PERINATAL MOOD & ANXIETY DISORDERS): 1-800-944-4773 OR WWW.POSTPARTUM.NET

 ### DOMESTIC VIOLENCE, ABUSE, AND ASSAULT
- NATIONAL DOMESTIC VIOLENCE HOTLINE: 1-800-799-SAFE (7233) OR TEXT "START" TO 88788
- RAINN (RAPE, ABUSE & INCEST NATIONAL NETWORK): 1-800-656-HOPE (4673)
- STRONGHEARTS NATIVE HELPLINE: 1-844-762-8483

 ### PARENTING & MATERNAL SUPPORT
- NATIONAL PARENT HELPLINE: 1-855-427-2736
- LA LECHE LEAGUE BREASTFEEDING HELPLINE: WWW.LLLI.ORG
- POSTPARTUM SUPPORT WARMLINE: 1-888-404-776

 ### SEXUAL & INTIMATE PARTNER HEALTH
- LOVE IS RESPECT (HEALTHY RELATIONSHIPS FOR TEENS & YOUNG ADULTS): 1-866-331-9474 OR TEXT "LOVEIS" TO 22522
- NATIONAL HUMAN TRAFFICKING HOTLINE: 1-888-373-7888 OR TEXT "HELP" TO 233733

 ### FINANCIAL & HOUSING SUPPORT
- NATIONAL HOMELESS HOTLINE: 1-800-569-4287
- WOMEN'S LAW HELPLINE (LEGAL HELP FOR WOMEN): WWW.WOMENSLAW.ORG

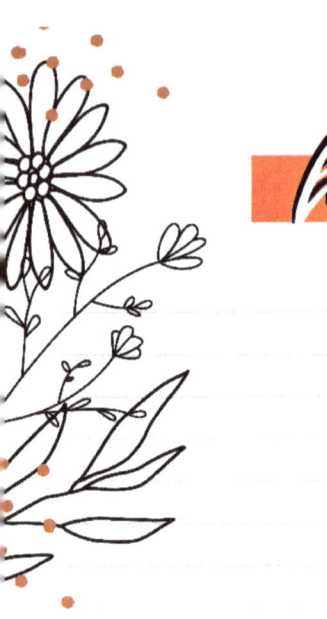 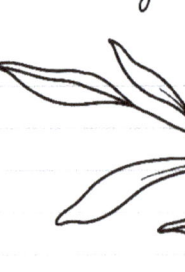

her NOTES

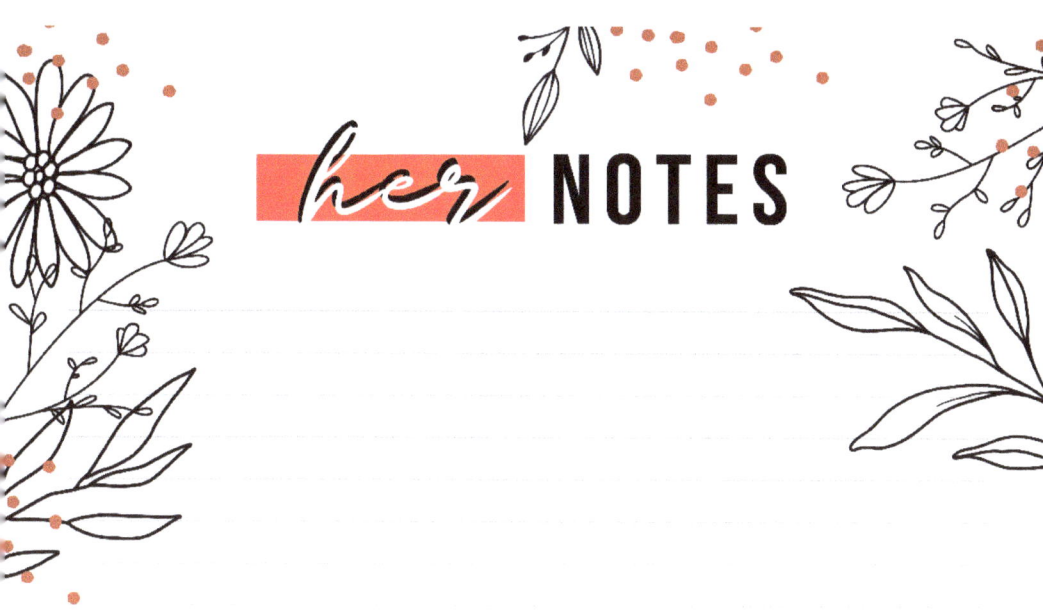

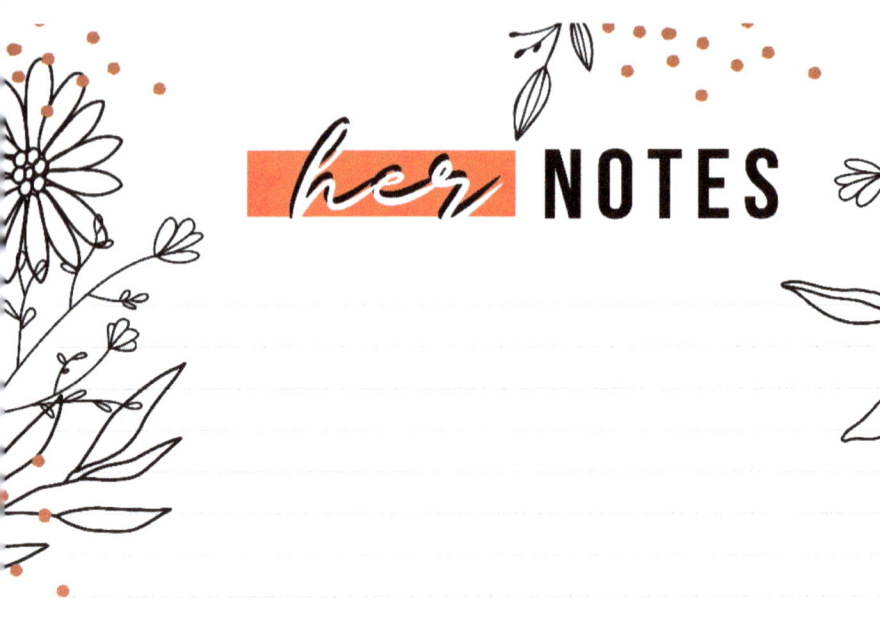

her NOTES

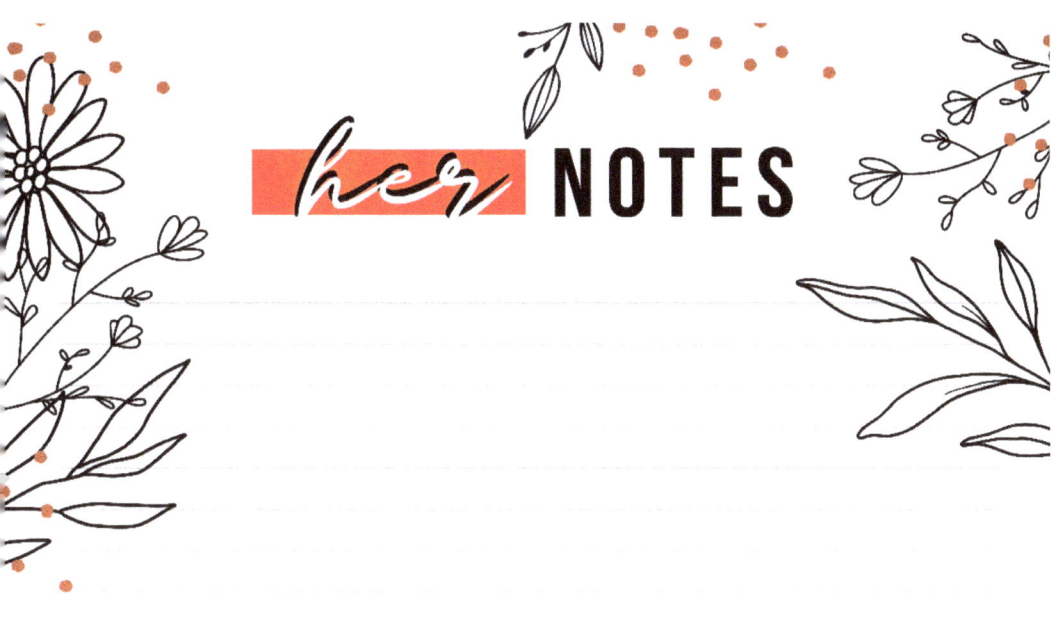

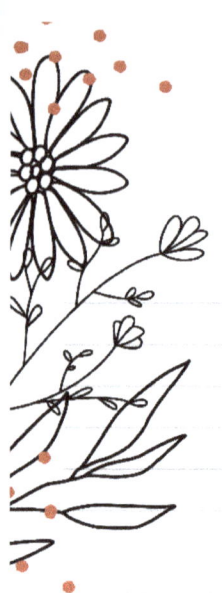 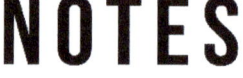 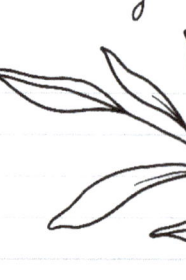

her NOTES

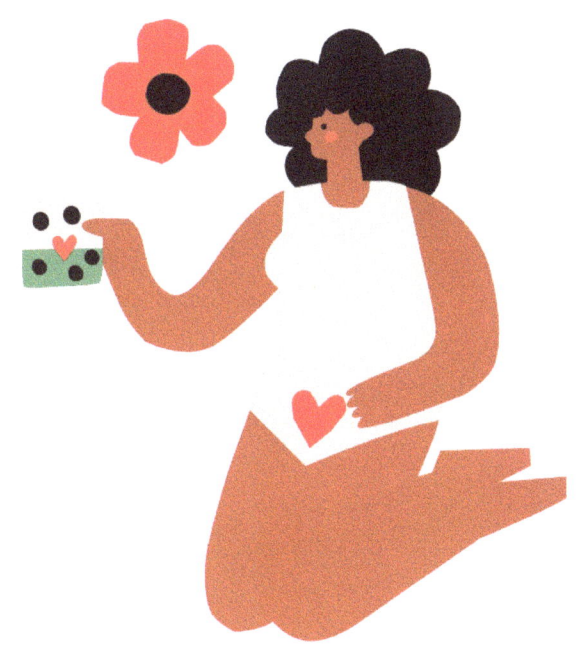

About The Author

Kirby Duncan is a mother, entrepreneur, and passionate advocate for holistic feminine wellness. As the founder of *YoniRx*, a brand dedicated to natural, microbiome-friendly solutions for women's health, Kirby has made it her mission to bridge the gap between traditional wisdom and modern science—empowering women to reclaim their well-being from the inside out. But this journey wasn't just professional, it was deeply personal.

Like many women, Kirby grew up without the full story when it came to feminine health. Her journey was marked by discomfort, confusing symptoms, and a cycle of quick fixes that never quite got to the root. It wasn't until motherhood (and the physical and emotional changes that came with it) that she began to uncover a deeper truth: true wellness isn't just about treating symptoms, it's about reclaiming connection with your body, your cycles, and yourself.

Through research, healing, and radical self-awareness, Kirby transformed her struggles into purpose and now helps other women do the same.

Losing a mother and grandmother to ovarian cancer further solidified Kirby's dedication to women's health. With three daughters to guide, the mission became clear: to create resources, products, and knowledge that would empower future generations to care for themselves in ways many of us were never taught.

Through *The Alchemy of Her*, Kirby shares the tools, insights, and rituals that helped her transform her own feminine health, offering every woman the opportunity to reconnect with her body's natural rhythm.

And the journey doesn't stop here. Look out for *The Alchemy of Her Daughter,* a companion guide for anyone raising a girl—mothers, fathers, aunties, teachers, bonus parents, and mentors. It's designed to help you navigate the changes, conversations, and milestones that shape her into a strong, confident, and prepared young woman.

This book doesn't just teach what's happening to her body—it offers the language, tools, and wisdom to help her understand herself, feel empowered in her choices, and walk into womanhood with grace and courage.

Raising her is a sacred task. Let's get it right, together.

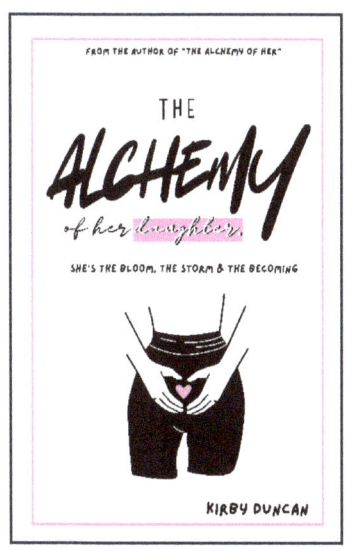

Let's Connect

Thank you for reading The Alchemy of Her. This book was just the beginning.

To stay connected, receive updates, and be the first to know about new releases, offerings, and holistic tools for your journey:

Follow Along Online
Instagram: @yonirxco / @kirbyaduncan
TikTok: @yonirxco / @kirbyaduncan
Facebook: YoniRx / Kirby uncan
Website: www.yonirx.co

Write to Me
I'd love to hear your story. If this book moved you, tag me on socials, send a message, or leave a review. Your voice matters.

With love,

Kirby Duncan

Sources & Citations

Hormonal Health & Reproductive Wellness

- Briden, Lara. Period Repair Manual: Natural Treatment for Better Hormones and Better Periods.

- Northrup, Christiane. Women's Bodies, Women's Wisdom: Creating Physical and Emotional Health and Healing.

- Romm, Aviva. The Adrenal Thyroid Revolution: A Proven 4-Week Program to Rescue Your Metabolism, Hormones, Mind & Mood.

- The American College of Obstetricians and Gynecologists (ACOG) - www.acog.org

- The Endocrine Society - www.endocrine.org

- National Institute of Environmental Health Sciences (NIEHS) - www.niehs.nih.gov

- The American Association of Naturopathic Physicians (AANP) - www.naturopathic.org

- National Institutes of Health (NIH) Women's Health - www.nih.gov/women

- PubMed & Clinical Research Studies on Women's Hormonal Health - www.pubmed.ncbi.nlm.nih.gov

Gut Health & The Microbiome

- Dr. Will Bulsiewicz, Fiber Fueled: The Plant-Based Gut Health Program for Losing Weight, Restoring Your Health, and Optimizing Your Microbiome.

- Dr. Robynne Chutkan, The Microbiome Solution: A Radical New Way to Heal Your Body from the Inside Out.

- National Institute of Diabetes and Digestive and Kidney Diseases (NIDDK) - www.niddk.nih.gov

- Harvard T.H. Chan School of Public Health - www.hsph.harvard.edu

- Dr. Mark Hyman, The Pegan Diet: 21 Practical Principles for Reclaiming Your Health in a Nutritionally Confusing World.

Menstrual Cycle Health & Period Support

- Clue App (Menstrual Health Research) – www.helloclue.com
- Flo Living – www.floliving.com
- Dr. Jolene Brighten, Beyond the Pill: A 30-Day Program to Balance Your Hormones, Reclaim Your Body, and Reverse the Dangerous Side Effects of the Birth Control Pill.
- The Fertility Awareness Method (FAM) – Research from Toni Weschler, Taking Charge of Your Fertility.
- The Association of Reproductive Health Professionals (ARHP) – www.arhp.org

PCOS, Endometriosis & Hormonal Disorders

- National Polycystic Ovary Syndrome Association – www.pcosaa.org
- Amy Medling, Healing PCOS: A 21-Day Plan for Reclaiming Your Health and Life with Polycystic Ovary Syndrome.
- Endometriosis Foundation of America – www.endofound.org
- Office on Women's Health, U.S. Department of Health & Human Services – www.womenshealth.gov
- Dr. Fiona McCulloch, 8 Steps to Reverse Your PCOS: A Proven Program to Reset Your Hormones, Repair Your Metabolism, and Restore Your Fertility.

Fertility, Birth Control & Pregnancy Support

- The American Society for Reproductive Medicine (ASRM) – www.asrm.org
- The Fertility Institute – www.fertilityinstitute.com

- World Health Organization (WHO) Research on Women's Fertility – www.who.int/reproductivehealth

- The Natural Cycles Birth Control App – www.naturalcycles.com

Menopause & Perimenopause

- The North American Menopause Society (NAMS) – www.menopause.org

- Dr. Mary Claire Haver, The Galveston Diet: A Menopause-Friendly Nutrition Plan to Balance Hormones and Reduce Symptoms.

- Dr. Christiane Northrup, The Wisdom of Menopause: Creating Physical and Emotional Health and Healing During the Change.

- Research on Phytoestrogens & Natural Hormone Replacement Therapy – www.ncbi.nlm.nih.gov

Libido, Sexual Wellness & Vaginal Health

- The American Sexual Health Association (ASHA) – www.ashasexualhealth.org

- Emily Nagoski, Come As You Are: The Surprising New Science That Will Transform Your Sex Life.

- The Journal of Sexual Medicine – www.jsm.jsexmed.org

- The Vaginal Microbiome & pH Balance Research – www.microbiomejournal.com

- The Women's Health Initiative (WHI) Research on Hormones & Sexual Health – www.whi.org

Stress, Burnout & Cortisol Management

- Dr. Mariza Snyder, The Essential Oils Hormone Solution: Reclaim Your Energy and Focus and Lose Weight Naturally.

- Dr. Sara Gottfried, The Hormone Cure: Reclaim Balance, Sleep, Sex Drive & Vitality Naturally with The Gottfried Protocol.

- The National Sleep Foundation (NSF) – www.sleepfoundation.org
- Research on Cortisol & Adrenal Fatigue – www.hormone.org
- The Chopra Center Research on Mindfulness & Stress Reduction – www.chopra.com

Detoxification & Toxin-Free Living

- The Environmental Working Group (EWG) – www.ewg.org
- Research on Endocrine Disruptors & Xenoestrogens – www.endocrine.org
- The Clean Beauty Movement – www.cleanbeauty.com
- Dr. Alejandro Junger, Clean: The Revolutionary Program to Restore the Body's Natural Ability to Heal Itself.

Beauty & Body

- Romm, Aviva. *Hormone Intelligence: The Complete Guide to Calming Hormone Chaos and Restoring Your Body's Natural Blueprint for Well-Being.*
- Briden, Lara. *Period Repair Manual: Natural Treatment for Better Hormones and Better Periods.*
- The American Academy of Dermatology (AAD) – www.aad.org
- Environmental Working Group (EWG), *Skin Deep® Database* – www.ewg.org/skindeep
- Campaign for Safe Cosmetics – www.safecosmetics.org
- Endocrine Society Scientific Statements on EDCs – www.endocrine.org
- Mount Sinai Health Library – www.mountsinai.org/health-library
- Cleveland Clinic: Dry Skin & Skin Health Resources – my.clevelandclinic.org
- Linus Pauling Institute, Oregon State University: Micronutrients & Skin/Nail Health – lpi.oregonstate.edu

- National Institutes of Health (NIH) – Office of Dietary Supplements – www.ods.od.nih.gov

- PubMed Research on Omega-3s, Biotin, and Skin/Hair Health – www.pubmed.ncbi.nlm.nih.gov

- International Journal of Cosmetic Science – www.onlinelibrary.wiley.com/journal/14682494

- @lainanicolee on TikTok (How to Always Smell Good 101)

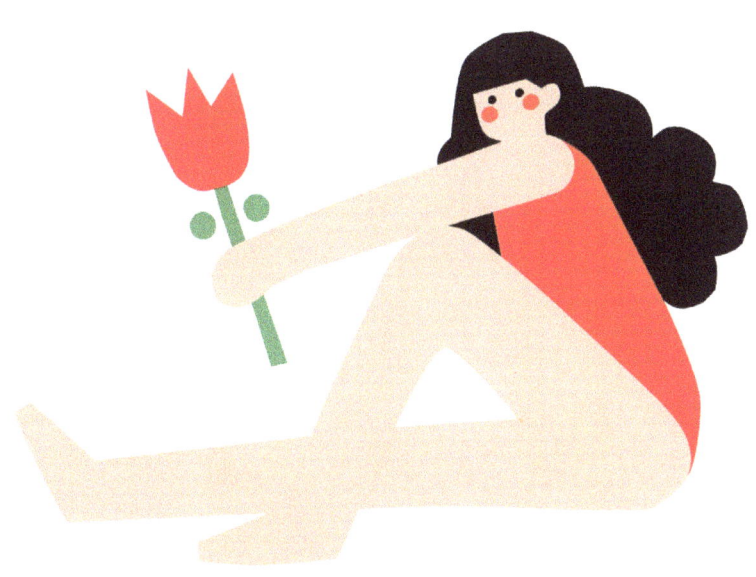

www.ingramcontent.com/pod-product-compliance
Lightning Source LLC
Chambersburg PA
CBHW052128030426
42337CB00028B/5065